Jane Fonda
Cooking for Healthy Living

RECIPES
Robin Vitetta

PHOTOGRAPHS
Joyce Oudkerk Pool

ILLUSTRATIONS
Jennie Oppenheimer

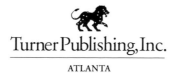

Turner Publishing, Inc.

ATLANTA

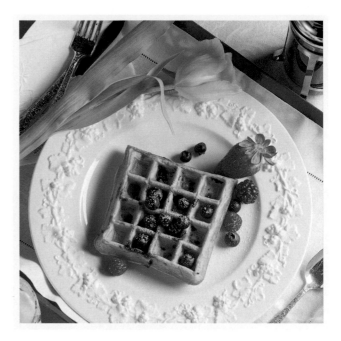

Published by Turner Publishing, Inc.

A Subsidiary of Turner Broadcasting System, Inc.

1050 Techwood Drive, N.W.

Atlanta, Georgia 30318

Library of Congress Cataloging-in-Publication Data:

  Fonda, Jane, 1937–

  [Cooking for healthy living]

  Jane Fonda cooking for healthy living/recipe writer, Robin Vitetta; photographer, Joyce Oudkerk Pool; illustrator, Jennie Oppenheimer. —1st ed.

  p. cm.

  ISBN 1–57036–293–9 (alk. paper)

  1. Cookery, American. 2. Nutrition. 3. Menus. 4. Diet.

  I. Vitetta, Robin. II. Title.

  TX715.F668 1996

  641.5973—dc20   CIP 96-15276

First Edition

10 9 8 7 6 5 4 3 2 1

Printed in United States of America

Back Cover: Colorful Sesame Chicken and Snow Peas in Apricot Sauce (recipe on page 140) is the main dish in a dinner (menu on page 129) that also includes a salad, pasta and cheesecake yet contains just 675 calories and only 8 percent calories from fat.

Above Right: Treat someone special to a beautiful breakfast of Very Berry Waffles (recipe on page 67) that is high in fiber and get their day off to a healthy start.

Produced by Weldon Owen, Inc.

814 Montgomery Street

San Francisco, California 94133

Separations by Colourscan, Singapore

Printed by R.R. Donnelley

Willard, Ohio

Distributed by Andrews and McMeel

A Universal Press Syndicate Company

4900 Main Street

Kansas City, Missouri 64112

Promoted by LaFonda Partners

340 Oswego Pointe Drive

Lake Oswego, Oregon 97034

A Note on Weights and Measures: All recipes include customary U.S. and metric measurements. Metric conversions are based on a standard developed for this book and have been rounded off. Measurements listed in the nutritional analysis have been rounded off as well. Unless otherwise stated, the recipes were designed for medium-sized fruits and vegetables.

*This book is dedicated with love to people who,
like myself, want to know how to cook healthy meals that
are easy to prepare, delicious to eat and good for you.*
— *Jane Fonda*

Contents

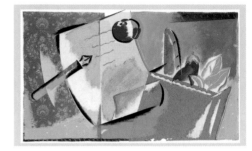

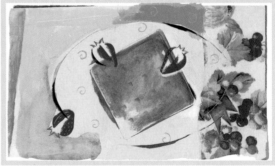

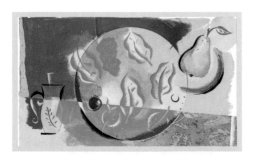

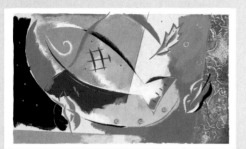

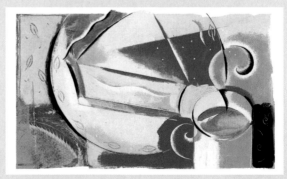

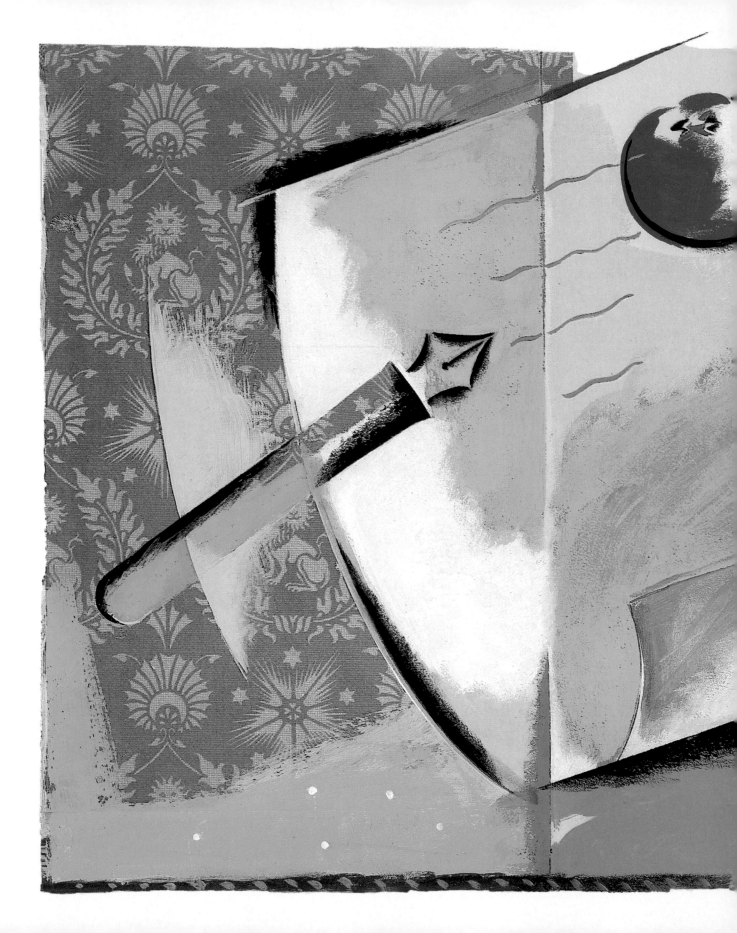

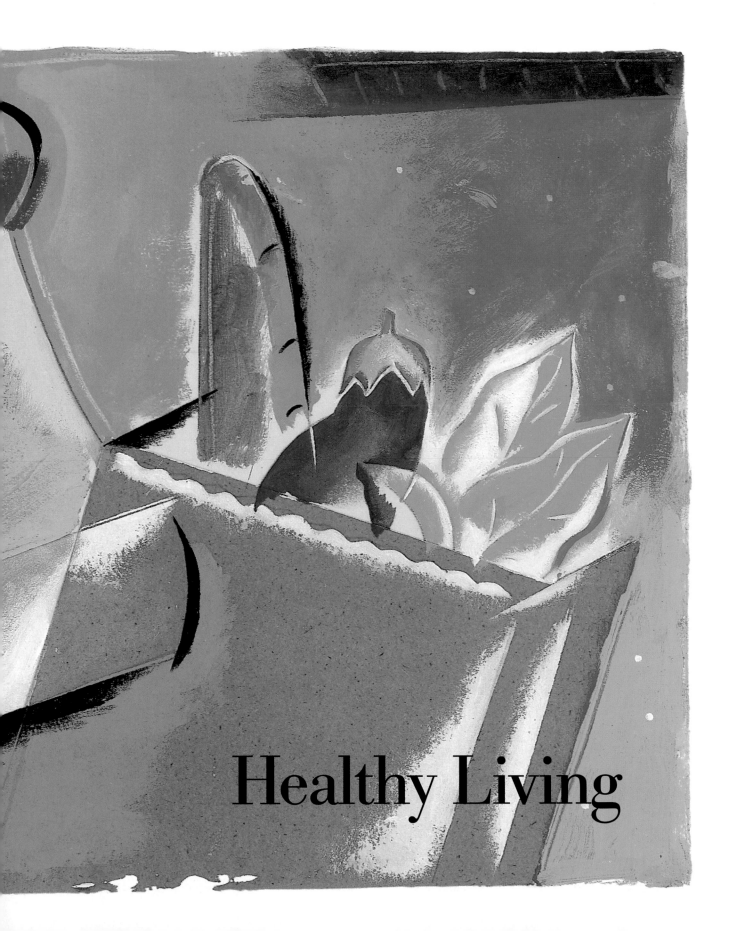

Healthy Living

Enjoying Healthy Living

Cooking for healthy living means planning meals that make use of fresh foods, which are prepared to retain their nutrients and maximize their flavors. It means savoring seasonal produce and experiencing nature's broad palette of colors and flavors. It means enjoying delicious, satisfying meals with attention and deliberation and not rushing absentmindedly through to the end. It means drinking water to lubricate your whole body. And, when combined with exercise, it means establishing and maintaining a metabolism that will let you eat more and weigh less.

Following these principles, you'll never have to diet and you'll never feel deprived. You'll eat wonderfully satisfying meals and you'll be in control of your weight. And you'll feel, act and look more healthy than ever before. In this introduction, I will share with you the nutritional principles and lifestyle habits that have made a profound difference in the quality and health of my life.

These introductory sections are intended to explain the sound nutritional principles behind the recipes and menus in this book. The recipes and menus have been developed in close collaboration with me by nutrition and cooking expert Robin Vitetta and a team of consultants to reflect my personal approach to healthy cooking and eating and to help you effortlessly adopt those principles.

First, however, I'd like to tell you about the paths in my life that have led me toward a greater awareness of what it means to eat healthily. I hope you'll find some parallels in your own experiences and take heart from the fact that, whatever your past, you *can* change the way you cook and eat, starting today.

It seems that whenever I read a good cookbook, it describes how the author grew up in a family that loved to cook, learned the basics by hanging around

the kitchen at his or her father's or mother's elbow, and ever since then has enjoyed a lifelong passion for cooking. None of these things were particularly true for me. When I was growing up, we always had someone who cooked for us, and the kitchen was never a very welcoming place.

One thing from my childhood has had a lasting influence on my health, and that is eating fresh, seasonal produce. My father, Henry Fonda, a midwesterner by birth and by nature, was an avid gardener. As far back as I can remember, he enjoyed growing his own vegetables and fruit.

Until I was 10, we lived on a sort of farm in the foothills of the Santa Monica Mountains overlooking the Pacific Ocean. It was the Second World War, food was rationed, and growing a Victory Garden was seen as an act of patriotism. At least to my young eyes, however, ours was more than just a garden. We had acres of vegetables and fruit trees and an enormous rabbit and chicken coop with individual pens for the laying hens, where their eggs would roll down into a trough to be gathered, still warm. To this day, I harbor a special fondness for fresh soft-boiled eggs.

It was on this farm, when he was not serving on a Navy destroyer in the Pacific, that my father taught me and my brother, Peter, about composting and how chicken droppings made the best fertilizer. I'm still proud that I can recognize rhubarb, asparagus and a host of other vegetables as their greenery first sprouts from the earth.

Toward the end of my father's life, he lived in the upscale Los Angeles enclave of Bel-Air. There, he transformed a portion of his manicured property into vegetable gardens that followed the French intensive method of raised beds, better suited to a smaller area. He grew many fruit trees and raised bees for their honey. He even built a sizable chicken coop where the roosters' crowing gave proof that, though he was now famous and was living fancier, Henry Fonda was still a product of the Great Plains, a farmer at heart, willing to press his luck with local codes that forbade livestock.

My father's love of gardening taught me to appreciate freshly grown produce and to pass this appreciation, as if by osmosis, on to my children. My daughter Vanessa, in particular, follows in her grandfather's steps, avidly tending vegetables in a tiny plot behind her home in Washington, D.C.

Though I had little childhood experience in the kitchen, for better or worse

How to Use This Book

COOKING FOR HEALTHY LIVING has been created and structured to make it as easy as possible for you to incorporate principles of healthy cooking and eating into your life. The following features work together to make that goal attainable:

✳ **Introduction.** Please read over pages 8–29 for a comprehensive yet easy-to-follow discussion of healthy cooking and eating, the basic principles of nutrition, meal and menu planning, shopping tips, weight loss and exercise.

✳ **Suggested Menus.** Each of the three chapters on breakfast (page 30), lunch (page 78) and dinner (page 126) begins with 21 menus for complete, healthy meals. Please use these to help you plan your next day, week or month of healthy eating. Following each chapter's Suggested Menus are the featured recipes, accompanied by a beautiful photograph of the finished dish. The last chapter, Completing the Meal (page 174), presents the recipes that round out the menus—the drinks, side dishes, dressings and desserts—plus basic recipes and healthy cooking techniques referred to throughout the book. To help in your planning, each recipe includes preparation and cooking times, along with tips on substitutions, preparation techniques and storage information. The ingredients lists and cooking methods are simple and to the point, written so that even the beginner cook can make the dish perfectly the very first time.

✳ **Nutritional Analyses.** Each menu and individual recipe includes a nutritional analysis to assist you in planning your personal healthy-eating goals.

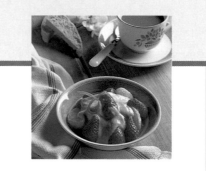

Poached Fruit with Cinnamon-Yogurt Topping
page 36

Example of a breakfast menu ———

Almond Biscotti
page 215

Where the recipe is located ———

Example of a recipe for completing the meal ———

Skinny Café Mocha
page 179

Nutritional analysis for the menu ———

Nutritional Analysis per Serving: Calories 364 (Kilojoules 1,529); Total fat 4g; Saturated fat 1g; Protein 11g; Cholesterol 27mg; Carbohydrates 73g; Sodium 196mg; Dietary fiber 3g; Calories from fat 9%

I've cooked a lot since the time, at age 24, I moved to France and married film director Roger Vadim, father of my gardener-daughter. I became a cookbook aficionada, reading everything from *The Alice B. Toklas Cookbook* to Escoffier's classic *Le Guide Culinaire*.

In early 1960s presupermarket France, shopping for groceries in my halting French, I must have seemed like a blind woman on a scavenger hunt. Vegetables were found only in the vegetable market, fish in the fish market, bread in the *boulangerie*. I remember the consequences of my first sortie to shop for a steak dinner. About five minutes into the meal, Vadim looked up and asked where I'd bought the meat.

"At the butcher," I said.

"Was there a horse's head over the door?"

In a flash, I realized what I'd done. Horse meat! I had cooked my favorite animal!

Though I never made that mistake again, I was a pretty adventuresome cook. The first time Vadim's ex-wife came over for dinner, I was really nervous. And why not? After all, she was Brigitte Bardot. I cooked *boudin noir*, "blood sausage." Maybe I was sending Brigitte a subliminal message. Neither of them suspected that I'd never seen a blood sausage in my life, much less cooked or eaten one.

My poor daughter took the brunt of my early efforts at healthy cooking. I so very much wanted to make sure she started her little life with the best possible nutrition. My bible at the time was health-food guru Adele Davis's *Let's Eat Right to Keep Fit*. When I weaned my daughter at four months, I put her on the formula Davis recommended: goat's milk, cranberry juice concentrate, a little yeast and *desiccated baby veal liver*. Needless to say, I had to make the hole in the nipple larger. When I eventually told a pediatrician what I had been feeding her and asked why she kept throwing up, he just stared at me in disbelief.

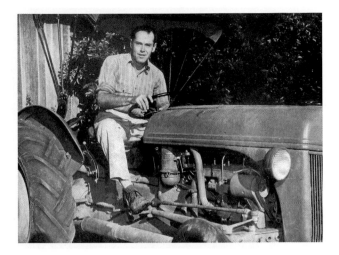

My father, Henry Fonda, shown here in a 1948 magazine photo, rides a tractor that was the pride and joy of his garden. He received the tractor for appearing on a Ford radio program. Known among his neighbors as the Compost King, he grew apples, oranges, berries and all the vegetables for our family's table.

My most memorable failure came at my daughter's third birthday party. I had followed, a recipe for a whole wheat birthday cake. As I walked from the kitchen carrying the cake with its candles aglow, I slipped. The cake shattered like a brick on the floor, necessitating a scramble to the bakery for the traditional, disgustingly gooey, undeniably delicious cake.

Since those Paris days, I've come a long way in my approach to healthy cooking and eating. Three and a half decades of dealing with the demands put on a professional actress to look good in a close-up after 15 hours on a soundstage have taught me sensible ways to eat meals that provide energy and vitality, are satisfying and tasty, and won't put on weight.

When I entered the health and fitness business in the late 1970s, I began working with nutritionists, doctors and sports physicians to learn the best ways to achieve maximum health through diet and exercise. As a mother, I learned the importance of serving well-balanced meals made up of a wide variety of fresh,

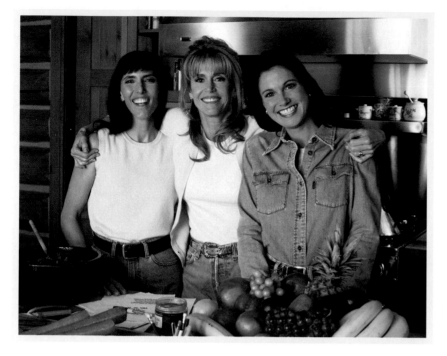

Karen Averitt (left) and I confer with Recipe Writer Robin Vitetta (right) in my Montana kitchen. Karen and I have worked together since the early 1980s. Several of her best recipes appear among the menus Robin developed for this book.

whole (nonprocessed) foods, cooked in ways that best retain their natural nutrients.

These days, I must admit, my fondness for really good food far exceeds my ability to cook it. Even if that weren't the case, there's not much time for me to do the cooking, since we entertain a lot and I, my husband, Ted Turner, and our frequent guests are usually outdoors right up until mealtime.

For that reason, the recipes in this book reflect not what I myself cook, but rather how I like to eat. I do, however, plan all our menus, and I am exceedingly fortunate to employ three talented people—in three different parts of the country where, depending on the season, we spend our nonworking time—who cook for us, following my dietary guidelines. These expert cooks have skillfully learned to adapt their regional styles to suit our desire for healthy meals.

In particular, I want to mention Karen Averitt, my longtime friend and associate who cooks for us when we are in Montana. When I ran a health spa she

managed the operation, prepared the meals and taught spa cooking. When Ted and I married, Karen and her musician-husband Jim Averitt moved to our ranch in Montana. Karen has learned to adjust the rather stringent spa menus to please my husband's Southern palate while keeping them healthy. She has developed a variety of wonderful lowfat ways to cook the fish, wildfowl and game that we catch, and the delicious free-range bison that we raise.

I have finally learned that healthy food doesn't have to be boring or strange. It can be so delicious that your family and friends won't even suspect that you're feeding them responsibly.

In this book, I want to teach you what I've learned about how to eat to maximize your health and energy; how to avoid overeating; and, for those interested in losing weight, how eating and exercise, like love and marriage, go together. You *can* make healthy eating and healthy living part and parcel of your life every day—morning, noon and night.

Understanding Wellness

We need networks of bike paths and jogging trails, neighborhoods that are designed for walking, safe streets that kids can play in, schools that encourage children to develop a lifelong love of physical activity, restaurant menus that list calories, and fun-filled activities that make young people not want to watch television."
—*Michael F. Jacobson, Ph.D.*
Executive Director, Center for Science in the Public Interest

Wellness has become a catchword in recent years for those of us interested in healthy living. Yet the concept isn't all that easy to grasp. That's because wellness isn't just the absence of illness and it isn't something you can achieve with a quick medical fix.

Wellness is a way of life. It takes into account the totality of your being: body, mind and spirit, both individually and in relation to each other. To achieve deep, true wellness, all three must be nourished.

This book seeks to help nourish the body. In doing so, it will also affect the mind and the spirit. And while you're thinking about life changes, why not also see what you can do in your community to bring about the changes Michael Jacobson envisions in the quote above, thus improving your own wellness and that of the people around you?

The Way We Eat

Human beings have many complex reasons for eating. It offers us a comforting social ritual, drowns our sorrows, fills the empty places in our heart or brings us pleasure.

Few of us give much thought to whether the sum of what we eat on any given day does what food is supposed to do: nourish us, providing the fuel and the building blocks our bodies need.

Whatever their function, each of the microscopic cells in our bodies is like a miniature factory. To do a good job, they require the best raw materials. Too often, these cells are plagued by pollutants—specifically substances called free radicals, which result from normal metabolic processes as well as from air pollution, cigarette smoke (ours or someone else's) and ozone. Free radicals cause cell damage and are a key factor in the aging process. Antioxidants—including vitamins C and E, beta-carotene and the mineral selenium—reduce the damaging effects. A healthy diet includes ample amounts of foods containing antioxidants.

The foods most of us eat on a daily basis, however, sorely lack these and other vital substances in sufficient quantities to keep our bodies working well. Instead, they include an excess of nutrients that slow us down and even damage us. Consider that 62 percent of the calories we put into our mouths comes from sugar, animal fats and alcohol, which have no fiber and little nutritive value. I like to refer to this as the Standard American Diet, with the all-too-fitting acronym SAD (see sidebar, page 14). The SAD diet accelerates the aging process by depriving our cells of the nutrients they need to regenerate and fight off the many environmental factors that bombard us daily.

Potentially Preventable Causes of Death in the United States

The SAD diet of processed-sugar breakfasts, fast-food lunches and dinners heavy on red meat is a recipe for disaster. As you can see in this chart, from the "Journal of the American Medical Association," the Standard American Diet is our biggest killer, with 300,000-plus deaths a year attributable to diet and lack of exercise.

[1990] SOURCE: J.M. McGinnis & W.H. Foege, *JAMA* 270,18,1993

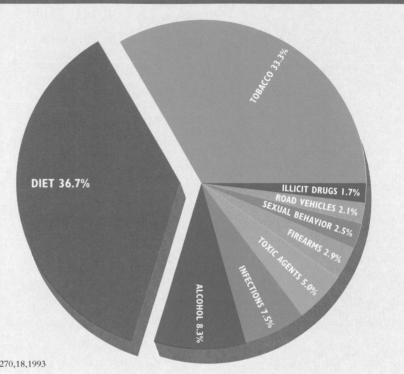

DIET 36.7%

TOBACCO 33.3%

ILLICIT DRUGS 1.7%
ROAD VEHICLES 2.1%
SEXUAL BEHAVIOR 2.5%
FIREARMS 2.9%
TOXIC AGENTS 5.0%
INFECTIONS 7.5%
ALCOHOL 8.3%

It's little wonder Americans tend to be unhealthy. Even the $35 billion fitness industry can't compete with this nation's always convenient 150,000 fast-food outlets and 4 million food vending machines, as well as a popular culture that promotes eating and lethargy over health and exercise. Too many of our children recognize sugary breakfast cereals more readily than fresh produce. We ride instead of walk, take elevators instead of stairs. We sit in front of our TVs an average of four hours a day—a figure even higher for the average teenager.

With medical costs ever rising and with so many things assaulting us that are beyond our immediate control, doesn't it make sense to take charge of the things we *can*? Wellness *can* begin at home—in what we cook and eat. It isn't difficult.

In fact, committing to a healthier way of eating can be easy and painless—and I'd like to show you how. It begins with learning a little bit more about the nutritional values of foods and how our bodies use them. With this knowledge, you can more easily plan your meals—a particularly important step for those seeking to lose weight and a step most often overlooked. Plan in hand, you can shop more sensibly. Using easy methods that most of us already know, you can cook food to maximize its taste and texture and preserve its nutritional value without adding calories or fat. Then, with the help of some simple strategies for modifying your behavior, you can actually eat that food in a different way that will bring you more pleasure, a greater sense of satisfaction and even, should you require it, weight loss.

Knowing Nutritional Basics

Here are the basic nutritional terms you'll need to understand when planning, shopping for, cooking and eating healthy meals: calories, protein, fat, saturated fat, cholesterol, carbohydrates, fiber and sodium. They form the basis for the nutritional analysis that accompanies every menu and recipe in this book. Use them as a guide in the long-term planning process.

Calories

For nutritional purposes, calories measure the amount of energy any given ingredient or finished recipe will provide you. We need a specific number of calories daily from food, depending on our size, weight, activity level and resting metabolism—the amount of energy a body must have simply to function. Eat more calories than you burn and you gain weight; eat fewer calories than you burn and you lose weight. One calorie is equal to 4.2 kilojoules—a term used instead of calories in some countries.

Protein

Present in seafood, poultry, meats, dairy products, legumes and grains, protein builds and repairs tissues and performs other essential functions. One gram yields about 4 calories (17 kilojoules) of energy, and a healthy diet will derive about 15 percent of daily calories from protein—the equivalent of about 6 ounces (185 grams) of seafood, poultry or meat. However, most Americans eat twice as much protein as they need; often, with it comes extra fat.

Fat

Everybody needs to eat some fat. It supplies us with fatty acids—essential substances that help move fat-soluble vitamins throughout our bodies—and also helps form and maintain the body fat we need for cushioning and insulation, stored energy, supple skin, healthy hair and some hormonal functions. One gram of fat yields 9 calories (38 kilojoules) of energy.

The trouble is, most of us eat far more fat than our bodies need, and too much of it in the form of saturated fat, instead of unsaturated fats that can decrease the overall level of blood cholesterol.

For the recipes in this book, I have aimed for an average of 25 percent of daily calories from fat; if you want to facilitate weight loss, choose those recipes with an even lower percentage.

You'll see that a few of the recipes derive more than 25 percent of their calories from fat. This doesn't mean you should avoid them. Rather, such recipes as Eggs Benedict (page 76) and Greek Salad (page 112) let you enjoy reduced-fat versions of high-fat dishes. As shown in the Suggested Menus in which such recipes are included, combine them with dishes that yield a lower overall fat content and choose lowfat recipes for your remaining meals that day.

Saturated Fat

No more than one-third of the day's total fat calories should come from saturated fat, present in animal proteins and in vegetable fats like palm and coconut oil. Saturated fat from animal proteins contains cholesterol, and all saturated fats increase the production of cholesterol by the liver—thereby raising total blood cholesterol levels.

Cholesterol

We could not live without cholesterol, which helps build hormones, cell membranes and nerve fiber sheaths. But our livers produce all we need.

When we eat too much saturated fat and animal protein and don't exercise enough, excessive cholesterol is deposited on arterial walls. The result: high blood pressure, stroke and heart disease. Experts agree that we should eat no more than 300 milligrams of dietary cholesterol a day.

Carbohydrates

Carbohydrates are the main source of energy in a healthy diet and should provide about 55 percent or more of our daily calories. They are classed into two categories: simple carbohydrates (sugars) and complex carbohydrates (starches). Like protein, one gram of carbohydrate yields about 4 calories (17 kilojoules).

When carbohydrates are digested, they become glucose—blood sugar. Glucose provides energy for the brain, the nervous system and the muscles, and must be available for a muscle cell to burn fat.

Simple carbohydrates are rapidly converted to glucose and absorbed into the bloodstream. In excess, they give an immediate energy burst, often swiftly followed by a precipitous drop. These so-called empty calories lack any other nutrients. Yet, avoiding them can be difficult, considering that 70 percent of the sugar in the average person's daily regimen is hidden in soft drinks, canned fruit, processed meat and commercial cereals. No more than 10 percent of total daily carbohydrate calories should come from sugars.

Foods high in complex carbohydrates—whole grains, pastas, cereals, breads, vegetables, legumes—are the fundamental wellness foods. Slowly digested, they supply steady energy, are chock-full of vitamins and minerals and are your best source of fiber.

Fiber

The body can't digest or absorb fiber, the residue from plant foods. Soluble fiber, which dissolves in water, slows down the digestion of carbohydrates, enabling their glucose to enter the bloodstream more slowly and yielding sustained energy. Soluble fiber also helps flush out cholesterol and toxins. It is abundant in oat bran, legumes and citrus fruits.

Insoluble fiber remains intact, absorbing water, expanding in the stomach and helping to pass food more quickly through the digestive tract while also sweeping out toxins. Insoluble fiber is found in whole grains, lentils, wheat bran, celery and beets.

Both kinds of fiber promote healthy, regular elimination. Experts recommend eating 25 grams a day.

Sodium

Sodium is widely misunderstood. Some of the mineral is needed by our bodies to help maintain proper levels of water, acids and bases and to regulate hormonal functions. However, we consume far too much of it. This comes not only through the salt we sprinkle on our food—about 2,200 milligrams per teaspoon—but also through its natural occurrence in many ingredients and its high levels in processed and snack foods. Most bodies eliminate excess sodium naturally; others tend to retain it. High levels of sodium lead to water retention, which can lead to high blood pressure. Drinking ample water daily helps flush out sodium. Experts recommend we eat between 1,100 and 3,300 milligrams of sodium a day.

The Food Pyramid

To help Americans easily understand the elements of a healthy daily diet, the United States Department of Agriculture and the United States Department of Health and Human Services jointly developed the Food Guide Pyramid, introduced in 1991. It clearly illustrates what proportion of your daily diet should be made up of each basic food group.

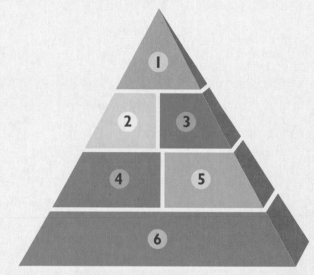

6 Breads, Cereals, Rice and Pasta: 6–11 servings

These abundant sources of complex carbohydrates, fiber and minerals provide most daily calories. One serving: 1 slice bread; $1/2$ cup (3 oz/90 g) cooked cereal, rice or pasta; $1/2$ cup (1 oz/30 g) ready-to-eat cereal; 1 pancake.

5 Vegetables: 3–5 servings

Excellent sources of vitamins, minerals and fiber, vegetables are also low in fat. One serving: 1 cup (2 oz/60 g) raw leafy vegetables; $1/2$ cup (3 oz/90 g) cooked or chopped raw vegetables; $3/4$ cup (6 fl oz/180 ml) vegetable juice.

4 Fruits: 2–4 servings

Fruits are excellent sources of vitamins A and C, folic acid and potassium; eaten whole, they are also high in fiber. One serving: 1 medium apple, banana or orange; $1/2$ cup (3 oz/90 g) chopped, cooked or canned fruit; $1/4$ cup ($1 1/2$ oz/45 g) dried fruit; $3/4$ cup (6 fl oz/180 ml) fruit juice.

3 Dairy Products: 2–3 servings

Milk, yogurt and cheese are good sources of protein, vitamins and minerals and are the best sources of calcium. One serving: 1 cup (8 fl oz/250 ml) milk; 1 cup (8 oz/250 g) yogurt; $1 1/2$ oz (45 g) cheese; 2 cups (16 oz/500 g) cottage cheese.

2 Proteins: 2–3 servings

Meat, poultry, fish, beans, eggs and nuts provide protein, B vitamins, iron and zinc. For the lowest fat, choose lean meats, skinless poultry, seafood, beans and lentils. One serving: 2–3 oz (60–90 g) cooked seafood, skinless poultry or lean meat; $1/2$ cup ($3 1/2$ oz/105 g) cooked dried beans; 1 egg.

1 Fats, Oils and Sweets: use sparingly

It is difficult to avoid some fats and sugars present naturally in foods. You can avoid consuming candy, cooking fats and foods processed with added sugar.

Planning Meals

With the knowledge of how basic nutrients make up a healthy daily diet and the serving numbers recommended on the Food Pyramid (see page 17), you can begin to plan your meals. Planning serves several useful purposes.

First, it lets you map out precisely what you will eat, ensuring a healthy balance of foods. Planning also provides you with a good shopping list, compiled from the ingredient lists of the recipes you plan to make. Not only will that list make shopping more convenient and economical, but it will guard against impulse buys of less healthy foods. If you are trying to lose weight, planning will help you reinforce your self-discipline.

Planning also helps you ensure another important aspect of healthy eating: variety. None of us can possibly manage to eat every single nutrient we need every single day. What is more important is to eat a varied diet that, over several days or a week, provides the full range of vitamins and minerals along with the more basic nutrients. Planning is the key to building variety into our diets.

Recognizing the importance of planning, 21 Suggested Menus lead off each of the next three chapters in this book to help you plan your meals for several weeks.

Breakfast

Breakfast is the perfect start to a day of healthy eating. Never skip it. If you do, or if you eat an inadequate breakfast, by late morning your energy will start to flag, and there's a good chance, unless you've thought to bring along a healthy snack, you'll try to pick yourself up with more coffee or a sugary treat.

A good breakfast featuring sufficient complex carbohydrates will digest slowly, gradually raising your blood sugar level and supplying steady energy. You should also include a small amount of protein, most conveniently in the form of milk or yogurt. This also supplies essential calcium and additional carbohydrate energy from milk sugar, or lactose. Those of us who have trouble digesting lactose can substitute soy milk.

Because eating for healthy living doesn't mean sacrificing all of your pleasures and giving up every habit, we've included coffee and tea on the Suggested Breakfast Menus (beginning on page 32). Whether or not they contain caffeine is your choice. A small glass of fruit juice, also listed with most breakfasts, is a good way to obtain a fruit serving.

Right: A wedge of Green Pepper-Corn Frittata, half an English muffin and a Strawberry-Banana Shake make up a well-planned breakfast (menu on page 35) that fulfills grain, protein, vegetable and fruit servings in only 383 calories for the complete meal.

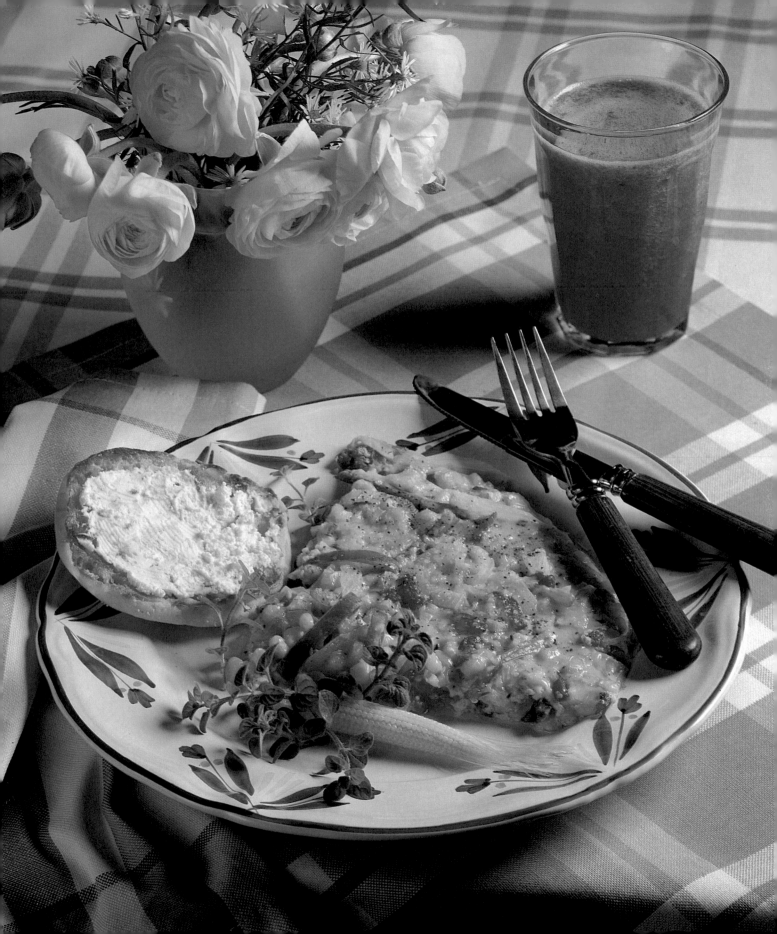

Snacks as Good Food

Many nutritionists sing the praises of dividing up the traditional three meals into several smaller meals eaten throughout the day. That isn't very practical for most people. But it is a good idea to have small portions of easy, healthy between-meal snacks on hand to stave off hunger, provide extra energy and help you avoid overeating later.

Here are some suggestions:

✳ Have a bowl of washed seasonal fruit always available on your counter or table.

✳ Prepare carrot and celery sticks, raw cabbage and Belgian endive (chicory/witloof) and have them ready to eat in the refrigerator.

✳ Pop air-popped popcorn.

✳ Carry salt-free rice cakes for coffee breaks.

✳ Cook your own baked tortilla chips (recipe on page 115) instead of buying salty commercial ones.

✳ Bake an extra potato for a snack (good-quality potatoes are delicious plain at room temperature).

✳ Drink a Smoothie (recipe on page 176) when you feel you must have something sweet.

✳ Substitute nonfat yogurt or Raspberry Sherbet (recipe on page 224) for ice cream snacks.

✳ Drink a glass of water when you feel hungry.

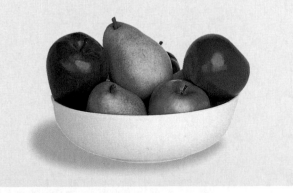

Lunch

Lunch is the best time to fill your daily protein requirements, accompanied by a variety of complex carbohydrates. Soup makes an especially satisfying lunch that meets your protein and carbohydrate needs while being lower in calories than solid foods—provided the soup has been defatted and made without cream or butter. Properly seasoned with herbs or spices, it won't be high in sodium, either. Because soup is usually hot, we tend to eat it more slowly than solid foods and wind up feeling full with a small portion.

If you work away from your home and don't have access to a cafeteria or restaurant that offers a good salad bar and other healthy selections, try brown-bagging it. Many of the lunch menus in this book pack easily. You'll need a wide-mouthed vacuum bottle for soup, cooked proteins, pasta or grains; an airtight container for salads or sandwich fillings; and a smaller container for dressing. Pack bread separately, building your sandwich at the last minute so it won't get soggy. Brown-bagging should save you time, too, providing a few extra minutes to take a midday walk or to have a workout at a nearby gym!

As you can see from the menus in this book, I don't favor fruit salad as the lunch main course. Such a concentration of sugars, even though they are natural ones, will give you quick energy but leave you drooping by midafternoon. If you are eating out and fruit salad is the only healthy option on the menu, have it with some protein—such as lowfat or nonfat cottage cheese or yogurt—and some complex carbohydrates for more sustained energy.

However, because people often have trouble including enough fruit in their diets, especially in winter, a piece of fruit and fruit juice are listed with most of the Suggested Lunch Menus (beginning on page 80). You may want to save the fruit for an afternoon snack. Drinking fruit juice with lunch, as with breakfast, is a good way to increase your fruit intake. Several of the menus suggest mixing fruit juice with seltzer water. This refreshing combination provides the bubbles of a soda without the caffeine.

Dinner

Although you can't always control when you eat at night, it's best not to eat dinner too late. In a well-publicized study, a group of people ate one 2,000-calorie (8,400-kilojoule) meal a day as either breakfast, lunch or dinner. Those who ate breakfast lost weight, those who ate lunch maintained their weight, and those who ate dinner gained weight.

Dinner should emphasize complex carbohydrates, with proteins used in small portions—almost like a garnish. Because they are bulky and take longer to digest, complex carbohydrates leave you feeling more satisfied—and less likely to snack later. Some researchers also think that they trigger the release in the brain of serotonin, a chemical that, among other functions, has a soothing effect, promoting better sleep. (It is interesting to note that the much-touted prescription drug Prozac helps the brain maintain levels of that same chemical.)

The Suggested Dinner Menus (beginning on page 128) all include dessert. Desserts do not have to be sinful to be delicious. Many of the desserts in this book are healthier versions of traditional sweets and others feature fruit as a main ingredient. While you may not want dessert every evening, when you do, these suggestions provide new options for a healthy ending to a meal.

No drinks are listed with the dinner menus and water is shown in the accompanying photographs.

The Importance of Water

We need to drink eight 8-fluid ounce (250-milliliter) glasses of water—not just liquids but pure water—every day. Too few of us do, and we take water so much for granted that we often fail to recognize the signs that we need it. We might feel sluggish or hungry when, in fact, we are dehydrated.

I cannot stress to you what a difference it can make to the way you feel to remain hydrated throughout the day.

Following my husband's example, at the beginning of 1994 I made a New Year's resolution to drink all the water I really needed. I carry with me a tall plastic bottle and make a point of drinking from it regularly over the course of the day, so that by bedtime it is empty. Every morning I refill the same bottle from a 5- or 10-gallon bottle of water.

I now feel less hungry throughout the day, especially when I drink a glass or two before a meal. My skin and hair are less dry. And I can see that water has a natural diuretic effect, largely eliminating fluid retention and bloating.

I find that it's easier to keep my water always with me if I carry my bottle in a holder with a shoulder strap. You'll find these everywhere now.

There are many other strategies you can use. Have a glass each morning in place of that second cup of coffee. Substitute it for an afternoon soda, adding a slice of citrus fruit. In your car, take a sip at every red light.

There are many strategies, once you think of water as liquid breath. Keep it flowing through you, moistening and cleansing your body.

Shopping Wisely

I remember once telling Katharine Hepburn how good her cooking was. She replied, in her inimitable voice, "It's because I know how to shop!" Experienced cooks firmly believe that knowing how to shop is essential to cooking tasty meals. A wise shopper can pick the best-quality ingredients, with the best taste, texture and nutritive value—at the best cost. Here are my tips:

✳ **Buy locally produced food.** That sounds like a simple statement, but there's a complex truth behind it best expressed in the book *Eight Simple Steps to the New Green Diet* by Mothers & Others for a Livable Planet: "The average mouthful of food travels 1,200 miles from farm to factory to warehouse to supermarket to our plates. In comparison, food available from local farms is almost always fresher, tastier, and closer to ripeness. . . . And, because it isn't being shipped long distances, local food is less likely to have been treated with post-harvest pesticides."

✳ **Develop sources.** Learn where you can buy the best quality and selection of fresh herbs, spices, dried beans and peas, rice, whole-grain cereals and breads.

✳ **Seek out organic products.** Organic foods are better for us and the environment. Organic fruits and vegetables are grown without pesticides or chemical fertilizers. Organic or free-range meats and poultry are raised without antibiotics or growth hormones.

Ask around for the best organic food market near you. Support organically grown foods and the people who produce and sell them so there will be a bigger demand, which will result in higher production and lower prices. If buying organic is not an option for you, don't feel any guilt about disregarding this tip. Just be very sure to wash produce well, scrubbing the fruits and vegetables you'll be eating, peels and all, to remove any traces of chemicals.

✳ **Seek out seasonal produce.** Again, I want to quote *Eight Simple Steps to the New Green Diet*: "Out-of-season produce is extravagant, because it is so amazingly energy-intensive. It costs about 435 calories [1,830 kilojoules] to fly one five-calorie [21-kilojoule] strawberry from California to New York. Out-of-season produce is also more likely to have been imported, possibly from a country with less stringent pesticide regulations than the U.S. Eating frozen fruits and vegetables, especially from local producers, is your very best option during the winter months. Frozen foods retain much of their nutritional content, in addition to cutting energy costs."

✳ **Patronize a service butcher.** If you cannot find a source for naturally raised meat or poultry, at least find a market where you can buy your meat fresh. Ask the butcher to cut it to order, and request that all excess fat be trimmed away.

✳ **Consider game.** Though I am not a vegetarian, I eat meat only in small portions, and for the most part, my family gets animal protein from elk, deer, bison and game birds. Game has far less fat and no chemical additives. Bison, for example, is lower in fat and cholesterol than chicken or turkey.

When You Must Substitute

The numbers below demonstrate why lowfat products are so helpful in creating healthy meals. When you must substitute other products, be sure to read product labels and adjust your nutritional analysis accordingly.

	CALORIES	TOTAL FAT	SATURATED FAT	CHOLESTEROL	SODIUM	CALORIES FROM FAT
For 8 fl oz/250 ml:						
Whole Milk	150	8 g	5 g	33 mg	120 mg	49%
Lowfat (2%) Milk	121	5 g	3 g	18 mg	122 mg	35%
Nonfat Milk	86	0 g	0 g	4 mg	126 mg	5%
For 8 oz/250 g:						
Lowfat Plain Yogurt	144	4 g	2 g	14 mg	159 mg	22%
Nonfat Plain Yogurt	127	0 g	0 g	4 mg	179 mg	3%
For 1 tablespoon:						
Unsalted Butter	102	11 g	7 g	31 mg	2 mg	99%
Salted Margarine	101	11 g	2 g	0 mg	134 mg	99%

✴ **Shop along the supermarket's walls.** Concentrate on fresh produce and on lowfat or nonfat dairy products, seafood, poultry and meats—all products commonly displayed along the walls. Go for a variety of produce colors, since each one offers different nutritional value. Most important are dark greens such as broccoli and cabbage, reds such as bell peppers and tomatoes, and yellows and oranges like cantaloupes, carrots and winter squashes.

✴ **Buy fresh produce at frequent intervals.** Try not to buy too much fresh fruit and vegetables at any one time. They begin to lose half their vitamin C after two or three days in the refrigerator, and even more quickly at room temperature.

✴ **Buy any frozen foods last.** To keep these in the best condition, put them in your cart just before you go to the checkstand.

✴ **Avoid empty calories.** Shop with an eye toward getting the most nutritive bang for your buck and your calories. This means avoiding processed foods, which usually cost more and are far higher in fat, sugar and salt than fresh foods.

✴ **Make a list.** Have a list to help you avoid impulse buying, especially when you get in the aisles where soft drinks, sweets and processed foods are stocked.

✴ **Learn to read labels.** Packaged products now carry labels that give all the pertinent information on nutrition content. A careful look at the ingredients list of a packaged product will also tip you off to the presence of monosodium glutamate, preservatives and other chemical additives.

✴ **Don't shop when hungry.** You'll make a wiser purchase, and spend less, if you shop on a full stomach. Drink some water before entering the market. If you still feel hungry, pick up a banana, a small pack of brown rice cakes or some other healthy snack and eat it while you shop. (Needless to say, save the peel or wrapper and tell the cashier to ring it up.)

Eating to Lose Weight

Like many women, I have not always had a healthy relationship with food. Perhaps that is why, today, I feel such sweet pleasure at being able to eat normally, healthily and without anxiety. I can do this because I have studied the effects different foods have on the body, I have learned the physiology of weight gain, and I have discovered, sometimes through hard experience, just how counterproductive dieting is. I've also worked on developing positive mental health.

There was a time not so long ago when the phrase "eating to lose weight" would have seemed an oxymoron. Losing weight meant not eating. In those days, I would starve myself, sometimes eating fewer than 500 calories a day and thinking even that was too much. I remember saying to anyone who commented on my radically restricted eating habits, "If I even eat an apple, I will put on weight."

I was right. My body was so starved that it burned muscle tissue to get the energy it needed. Because of the loss of muscle tissue, I had a very low metabolism. Anything I ate would be hoarded by my body as fat.

Today, I eat normal amounts of a wide variety of foods. Had I known sooner what I know now about how to avoid counterproductive dieting, how much easier and healthier my life would have been.

Consider the word *diet*. It derives from the Greek *diaita,* meaning "manner of living." That's what a weight-loss program should be: not some on-again off-again, feast-and-famine seesaw but a permanent, balanced, sustainable, metabolism-raising way of life.

Why Humans Store Fat

The roots of many people's weight problems may be found in evolution. Ten thousand years ago, humans lived as hunter-gatherers, moving with the seasons, searching constantly for adequate food supplies. The foods most reliably available were carbohydrate-rich vegetables and fruits. As a result, the human body did not need to develop a capacity for storing within itself large amounts of carbohydrates.

Meat was far more difficult to obtain. It would be eaten immediately, since meat was harder to store. Long periods of time might go by, especially during winter, when there would be no available fat, a crucial source of energy. We adapted by developing the ability to store fat within our bodies.

Today, our bodies still have a limited capacity for storing carbohydrates and an unlimited capacity for storing fat. We are sedentary, eating diets high in fats and sugars. No wonder some 26 percent of Americans are clinically obese.

Healthy Eating Out

Restaurants

Good restaurants are accustomed to special requests and are happy to comply.

✳ **Order small, healthy portions.** Ask for a salad or soup (made without cream or butter) as your appetizer. Then order another appetizer as your main course.

✳ **Ask for salad dressing on the side.** If you need the taste of dressing, dip your fork before you spear some lettuce.

✳ **Make special requests.** Don't feel self-conscious about asking for food cooked without butter, cream, salt and MSG.

✳ **Have an entrée strategy.** Choose entrées that are broiled, steamed, roasted, poached or grilled. Ask for sauces on the side. Split one main course with a companion or eat half and take the rest home for another meal.

✳ **Don't make a big deal about food preferences.** It's always a drag when someone goes on about his or her diet. Quietly and gracefully relay your requests to the waiter.

Air Travel

It is perfectly possible today to eat healthy food on an airplane.

✳ **Phone ahead.** Most airlines offer healthier options such as lowfat, low-calorie, seafood, fruit and vegetarian meals. Call at least 6 and usually 24 hours ahead.

✳ **Pack your own meal.** With the help of airtight, resealable bags and containers, ice packs and lightweight insulated carriers, pack a delicious, healthy carry-on meal.

✳ **Eat moderately, drink lavishly.** Eat as little as possible without being hungry and drink a lot of water. At least one glass every hour helps offset the dehydration caused by cabin pressurization and will minimize jet lag. Avoid alcohol.

Fast Food

Here's how you can make the best of fast-food restaurants.

✳ **Take the fresh approach.** Whenever possible, stick to salad bars, choosing only fresh vegetables and fruits.

✳ **Request nutrition details.** Most fast-food chains have flyers that provide nutritional analyses. Look them over.

✳ **Choose obvious lowfat options.** Select a grilled chicken sandwich. Ask for no sauce. Avoid fried foods.

✳ **Create your own pizza.** Order thin-crust pizza by the slice with vegetable toppings and without cheese. Fresh-baked crust topped with sauce and vegetables is delicious.

✳ **Have a high-fiber breakfast.** Stick to whole wheat toast or pancakes—without butter or syrup. Avoid egg sandwiches, bacon, sausage and croissants. Choose only lowfat muffins.

Automobile Travel

Here are some ways to break the habit of eating in your car.

✳ **Keep water handy.** If you feel hungry or tired, take a swig from a water bottle.

✳ **Lock temptations in the trunk.** Put the groceries in the trunk, out of temptation's way.

Banquets and Parties

Help yourself with these strategies.

✳ **Special-order your food.** Call the restaurant, catering office or party planners at least 24 hours ahead and order a vegetable plate.

✳ **Don't linger around buffets.** Sip water and mingle!

✳ **Keep dessert away.** Put a coffee cup or glass right in front of you, so the waiter can't even set down a dessert plate.

Of course, a number of other factors also come into play, including genetics, low metabolism and simple lack of physical activity. It is clear that we have to take matters into our own hands, combining moderate exercise with sensible lowfat eating.

Why Not Dieting?

Scientists have come to believe in what is called the Set Point Theory, which asserts that within each of us is a sort of thermostat that kicks into action if our body suddenly loses too much fat, nitrogen and potassium, attempting to bring us back to our set point by increasing our appetite. It also causes the body to consume muscle tissue for the energy that should be coming from food, causing our metabolism to drop and diminishing our ability to burn the calories from the food we consume.

So what, then, does "eating to lose weight" mean? First of all, it means eating enough food to keep you from feeling hungry and deprived and your "thermostat" from kicking into fat-retaining mode. Then, to have energy and good health, we have to eat a wide variety of healthy foods, without eating more than our metabolism can "burn" as energy. In addition, we must try to maintain an appropriate amount of muscle mass to ensure a healthy metabolism.

Switching to a lowfat diet makes cutting calories a lot easier—particularly when you consider that a gram of fat has 9 calories (38 kilojoules), while a gram of protein or carbohydrate has just 4 calories (17 kilojoules). You can eat a greater volume of lowfat food without risking weight gain.

However, don't think that, just because something is "fat-free," we can eat all we want. Always bear in mind that *calories do count*, whether from fat or from fat-free foods. If we eat more calories than we burn, they will be stored as fat no matter what their source.

Strategies for Eating Less

* **Keep a food diary.** Write down everything to see how much you eat without being aware of it.
* **Measure portions.** Measure the food you eat until you have internalized what correct portions look like—and how you feel after eating them.
* **Drink water.** Have a large glass before every meal.
* **Serve food on smaller plates.** Smaller portions will appear proportionately bigger.
* **Eat slowly.** It takes our brains about 20 minutes from the time we start eating to register that hunger has been satisfied. Eat more slowly, and you'll consume less food in that time. Take small bites, chew each at least 20 times, and pause between bites.
* **Don't let yourself get hungry.** Notice the times of day when your energy tends to flag and make sure you have a healthy, lowfat snack close at hand.
* **Do something else instead of eat.** When you feel the urge to eat and it's not mealtime, try to do something active like taking a brisk walk.
* **Don't eat when feeling anxious.** Learn ways to keep tension at bay. Relax and breathe deeply until the feeling passes. Yoga is a good way to handle tension and anxiety.
* **Be easy on yourself.** Everyone lapses from time to time. If you really crave a cheeseburger, have one. But then adjust what else you eat that day or the next. Don't let a little lapse turn into a relapse.
* **Remember: You're in control.** If you feel there is some vague authority figure saying, "You shouldn't eat this" and "You're bad if you do," you may react by overeating to spite that voice. Instead, relax, breathe deeply and take back control.
* **Make meals pleasurable occasions.** Set a pretty table. Light candles. Play music with a slow tempo to set your eating pace. Talk. The more enjoyable a meal, the more slowly you will eat.

Eating and Exercise

I've said it before, but here it is once again: For sustainable weight loss, you must burn more calories than you consume. Nutritionists estimate that an average active woman can lose weight eating 1,200 to 1,300 calories (5,040 to 5,460 kilojoules) a day and maintain her weight eating 1,600 to 1,900 calories (6,720 to 7,980 kilojoules) a day; the average man can lose weight eating 1,700 to 1,800 calories (7,140 to 7,560 kilojoules) daily and maintain his weight eating 2,000 to 2,400 calories (8,400 to 10,080 kilojoules). To achieve or maintain your desired weight (assuming your idea of desired weight is reasonable), you should eat within those calorie amounts and establish a regular program of physical activity.

Go for the Burn—the *Metabolic* Burn

By eating healthily and increasing the amount of exercise you do, you can raise your metabolism, reversing the vicious cycle of yo-yo dieting.

Think of your metabolism as, in part, the internal combustion that occurs in the cells of your body when digested fats, proteins and carbohydrates are "burned" to create energy, measured in calories. If we eat more calories than we burn, they will be stored as fat.

Sixty to 75 percent of the calories we burn each day are used to keep the body functioning while we are awake but resting. This is called our *resting metabolic rate* (RMR). As we exercise or just go about our lives, we use our muscles and thereby increase our output of energy above our RMR. Muscle is *active* tissue, and the more muscle we have, the higher our metabolism will be and the more calories we will burn.

Muscle is denser and more bricklike than spongy fat. That's why we can lose 3 pounds (1.5 kilograms) of fat, gain 3 pounds of muscle, not show any weight loss on the scale, but find our pants have become loose.

In short, the more lean muscle your body has, the higher your metabolic rate will be and the greater the number of calories you will burn just being alive.

It might interest you to know that middle-age spread is only partly due to the tendency to be less active as we age. The other reason is because we lose 3 to 5 percent of our muscle tissue each decade after age 30. This results in a slowing of our resting metabolic rate—unless we consciously work to increase our lean mass through exercise.

Train for Strength

You can increase your metabolism by building and maintaining your muscles. That doesn't mean you have to become bulked up like a weight lifter; instead, it just requires strengthening and toning your body through training with light weights. Although this can't reverse age-related loss of muscle tissue, it can definitely slow that loss and even restore some lost muscle tissue. It also will ensure that you maintain a metabolism that lets you eat a proper diet without gaining weight. According to my friend Dr. Daniel

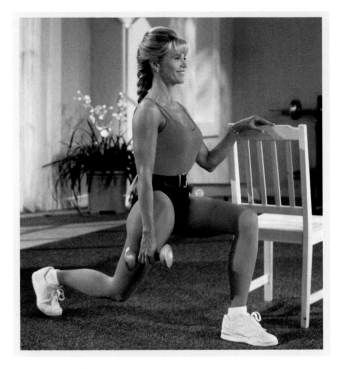

Kosich, it is likely that our resting metabolic rate burns at least 20 to 30 more calories (84 to 126 more kilojoules) a day for every 1 pound (500 grams) of muscle we add through strength training.

Let me say it again, because too many women (in particular) concentrate their exercise time on aerobics and forget about strength training: Muscles are very important for health as well as for aesthetic reasons.

Exercise Aerobically

Aerobic activity requires you to use your larger leg and arm muscles over a sustained period of time, which causes large amounts of oxygen-carrying blood to be pumped to your heart and your cells. Stored body fat can be burned only in the presence of oxygen, so it is this fat that is the source of energy during aerobic activity. To be effective, an aerobics program should entail a minimum of two 10-minute sessions a day or one 20-minute session a day, at least 4 days a week.

Put It All Together

Recent research suggests that the most effective way to lose body fat is to combine vigorous aerobic exercise with strength training, 2 to 4 days a week, and eat lowfat, moderate-calorie meals. Though you may consume more calories than a person who does not exercise, you will not gain weight and will have less fat and more muscle.

See the Resources Guide on page 240 for some exercise videos that can help motivate you and keep you on track.

One of the complaints about exercise I hear most often from people is that they don't have time. But there are many simple ways you can make exercise part of your daily routine. When shopping or running errands by car, park at the farthest corner of the lot. Don't take the car for nearby errands. Use stairs instead of elevators and escalators. Make dates to walk or bike after work. Most important of all, *write down exercise sessions as appointments.*

Erase Exercise Myths

Put to rest these *misunderstandings* about exercise.

✳ **Myth: You can spot-reduce.** Contrary to popular belief, it is basically impossible to exercise a specific part of your body to lose fat stored there. When you reduce by cutting calories or exercising more, fat is mobilized out of *all* the fat cells *all over the body.*

✳ **Myth: You can sweat off fat.** Sweating is water loss. This will quickly be replaced when you take a drink— which you must do for good health.

✳ **Myth: Muscles lock in fat.** Fat is subcutaneous— between skin and muscle—rather than between muscle and bone. An increase in your muscle mass through strength training will not somehow lock in your fat.

A Note on Eating Disorders

The eating disorders anorexia nervosa and particularly bulimia nervosa are common throughout the world today. I want to say a few words about the subject in the hope that someone for whom this information is relevant will read it and be helped.

Anorexia and bulimia are illnesses. They are not signs of moral weakness or character flaws. They are not who you are, but something that may have happened to you.

The illness may start in the most innocuous of ways—perhaps as a quick means of losing a few pounds. It progresses, however, until it takes on a life of its own, growing out of control and affecting your health, your moods, your perception, your work and your relationships. Left untreated, an eating disorder can shorten or even end your life.

Over the past few decades, science has shown that eating disorders, like heart disease, result from a complex pattern of risk factors. Researchers still don't know exactly which features are the causes of anorexia and bulimia and which are the results.

What is known, however, is that secrecy and anxiety are your worst enemies. Coming out of the closet about your illness is the first step to recovery, making it harder for you to continue facing your problem alone and harder for you to be covert—while, it is hoped, providing you with the support you need.

It isn't always easy for those close to you to be as understanding about eating disorders as you might like and need them to be. But it's important that you help them try. For that reason, I'd like to recommend "The Famine Within," an excellent, award-winning documentary on the subject (see page 240). I think this film could help those around you gain greater understanding and compassion for those who suffer from distorted body images and eating disorders.

More important still, anyone suffering from an eating disorder needs specialized professional help, starting with a complete medical, psychological and nutritional evaluation. A treatment team that includes a therapist, an internist and a dietitian will create a plan suitable for your particular needs and goals. Your therapist can advise you whether a local self-help group might also be worthwhile for you to join.

How recovery is defined, how long it should take and how difficult it will be all vary from person to person—and, to some extent, among treatment programs. "Bulimic patients treated with cognitive-behavioral therapy or with antidepressant medication often stop or greatly reduce their binging within four to six months, with a low rate of relapse over time," says Janice M. Cauwels, author of "Bulimia: The Binge-Purge Compulsion." "But bulimia nervosa is a closed circle in which distortions and miseries lead to severe, imbalanced dieting that causes binge-purging that aggravates the distortions and miseries. Short- or long-term individual, group, family or feminist therapy—or even hospitalization—may help some patients break this cycle at a different point." See the Resources Guide on page 240 for the names of helpful organizations.

With treatment, a bulimic will learn to recognize and change the thoughts and behaviors that trigger a binge, to express feelings and handle stress better, and to develop a stable, reliable eating structure in which no food is necessarily "forbidden." The further away from the binge-purge disorder the bulimic is able to grow, the easier it gets to eat in a healthy, anxiety-free way. In time, she (or he) can assume a more spontaneous relationship with a variety of foods and with normal weight.

I know because I did.

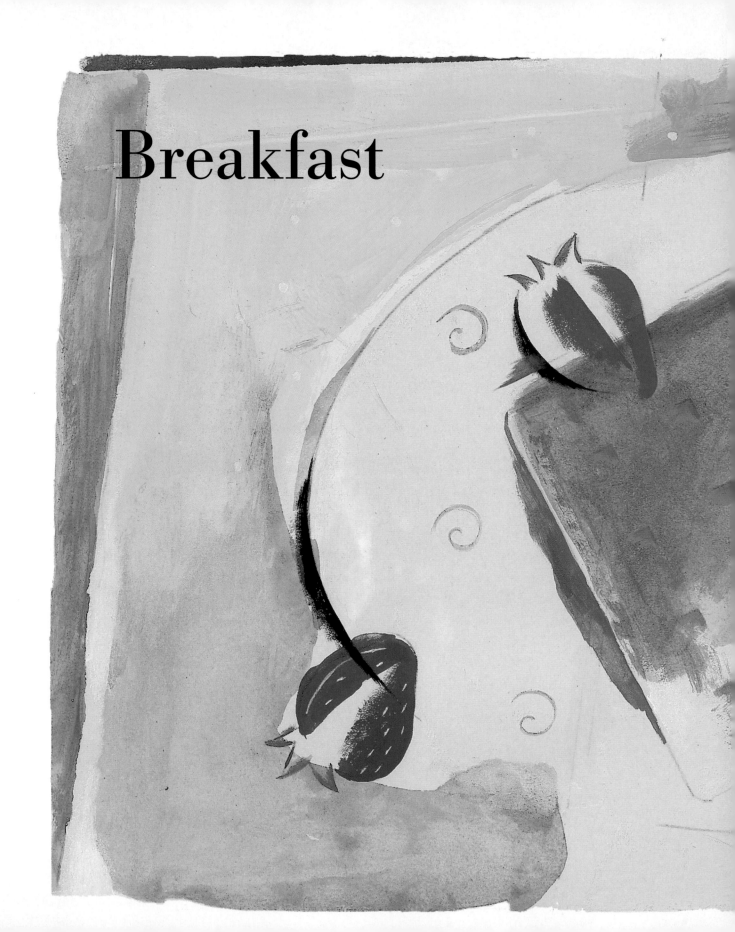

Breakfast

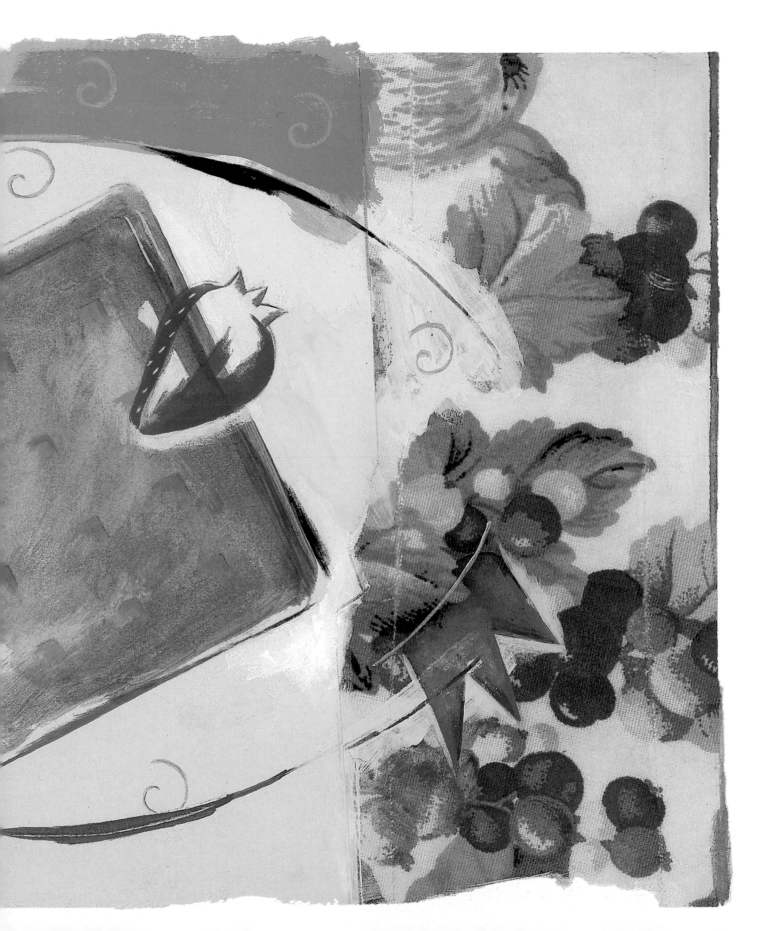

Suggested Breakfast Menus

Just as so many of our mothers told us years ago, breakfast is the most
important meal of the day. A well-balanced, satisfying breakfast featuring complex
carbohydrates and protein—in the form of whole-grain cereals or breads,
fresh fruits and nonfat dairy products—gives us the energy we need to begin
our work and to see the morning through without running the hazard of eating
a sugary or fat-laden snack that could derail our healthy eating goals. Use the menus
shown here and the recipes on the following pages as your guide to composing a
breakfast that not only meets your nutritional requirements but also is
easy to make and incomparably delicious.

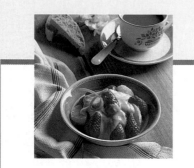

*Poached Fruit with
Cinnamon-Yogurt Topping*
page 36

Almond Biscotti
page 215

Skinny Café Mocha
page 179

Nutritional Analysis per Serving: Calories 364
(Kilojoules 1,528); Total fat 4g; Saturated fat 1g;
Protein 11g; Cholesterol 27mg; Carbohydrates 73g;
Sodium 196mg; Dietary fiber 3g; Calories from fat 9%

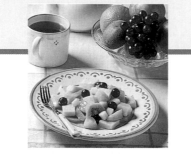

Almond Gelatin Squares in Fruit
page 39

*2 slices whole wheat toast
with 1 teaspoon margarine*

coffee or tea

Nutritional Analysis per Serving: Calories 496
(Kilojoules 2,085); Total fat 7g; Saturated fat 1g;
Protein 16g; Cholesterol 4mg; Carbohydrates 98g;
Sodium 469mg; Dietary fiber 9g; Calories from fat 12%

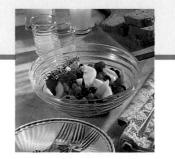

*Summer Fruit
in Rosemary Syrup*
page 40

Pumpkin Spice Bread
page 231

4 fl oz (125 ml) grapefruit juice

Nutritional Analysis per Serving: Calories 578
(Kilojoules 2,429); Total fat 8g; Saturated fat 1g;
Protein 9g; Cholesterol 53mg; Carbohydrates 120g;
Sodium 379mg; Dietary fiber 6g; Calories from fat 13%

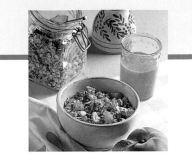

Hearty Granola
page 43

½ cup (4 fl oz/125 ml) nonfat milk

1 peach

Strawberry-Banana Shake
page 176

Nutritional Analysis per Serving: Calories 666 (Kilojoules 2,796); Total fat 12g; Saturated fat 2g; Protein 19g; Cholesterol 3mg; Carbohydrates 128g; Sodium 102mg; Dietary fiber 11g; Calories from fat 16%

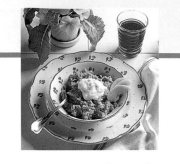

Apple-Raisin Oatmeal
page 44

4 fl oz (125 ml) cranberry juice

Nutritional Analysis per Serving: Calories 338 (Kilojoules 1,418); Total fat 3g; Saturated fat 1g; Protein 7g; Cholesterol 1mg; Carbohydrates 74g; Sodium 31mg; Dietary fiber 5g; Calories from fat 7%

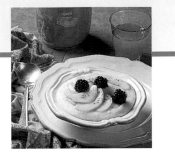

Hot Wheat Cereal with Gingered Peaches
page 47

4 fl oz (125 ml) apple juice

Nutritional Analysis per Serving: Calories 368 (Kilojoules 1,544); Total fat 1g; Saturated fat 0g; Protein 6g; Cholesterol 0mg; Carbohydrates 86g; Sodium 10mg; Dietary fiber 4g; Calories from fat 2%

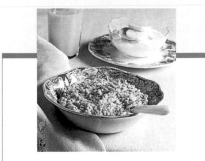

Irish Oatmeal
page 48

½ cup (4 oz/125 g)
nonfat plain yogurt with
½ banana

4 fl oz (125 ml) orange juice

Nutritional Analysis per Serving: Calories 352 (Kilojoules 1,480); Total fat 3g; Saturated fat 1g; Protein 15g; Cholesterol 2mg; Carbohydrates 68g; Sodium 642mg; Dietary fiber 6g; Calories from fat 8%

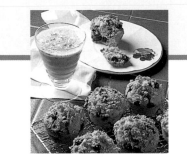

Blueberry Muffins
page 51

Sunshine Smoothie
page 176

coffee or tea

Nutritional Analysis per Serving: Calories 287 (Kilojoules 1,205); Total fat 4g; Saturated fat 1g; Protein 6g; Cholesterol 4mg; Carbohydrates 60g; Sodium 323mg; Dietary fiber 4g; Calories from fat 12%

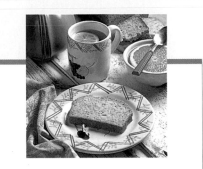

Banana Bread
page 52

½ grapefruit

coffee or tea

Nutritional Analysis per Serving: Calories 320 (Kilojoules 1,344); Total fat 1g; Saturated fat 0g; Protein 6g; Cholesterol 0mg; Carbohydrates 74g; Sodium 360mg; Dietary fiber 3g; Calories from fat 3%

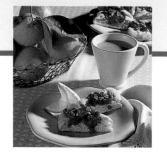

Cranberry-Pecan Scones
page 55

1 orange

Hot Cocoa
page 179

Nutritional Analysis per Serving: Calories 550 (Kilojoules 2,310); Total fat 9g; Saturated fat 2g; Protein 17g; Cholesterol 6mg; Carbohydrates 103g; Sodium 586mg; Dietary fiber 6g; Calories from fat 14%

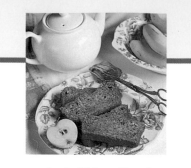

Apple-Walnut Bread
page 56

1 banana

coffee or tea

Nutritional Analysis per Serving: Calories 377 (Kilojoules 1,585); Total fat 7g; Saturated fat 1g; Protein 7g; Cholesterol 27mg; Carbohydrates 76g; Sodium 318mg; Dietary fiber 4g; Calories from fat 17%

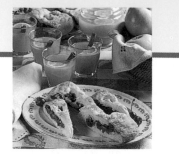

Cherry-Cheese Coffee Ring
page 59

1 apple

Hot Fruit Cider
page 180

Nutritional Analysis per Serving: Calories 553 (Kilojoules 2,324); Total fat 3g; Saturated fat 0g; Protein 12g; Cholesterol 3mg; Carbohydrates 123g; Sodium 299mg; Dietary fiber 6g; Calories from fat 4%

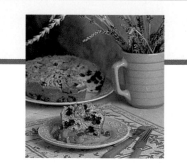

Blueberry Coffee Cake
page 60

Cranberry-Applesauce
page 212

coffee or tea

Nutritional Analysis per Serving: Calories 541 (Kilojoules 2,273); Total fat 4g; Saturated fat 1g; Protein 9g; Cholesterol 3mg; Carbohydrates 120g; Sodium 387mg; Dietary fiber 5g; Calories from fat 7%

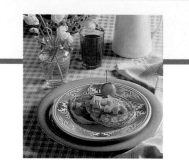

*Oat-Buttermilk Pancakes
with Honey-Fruit Sauce*
page 63

4 fl oz (125 ml) cranberry juice

Nutritional Analysis per Serving: Calories 440 (Kilojoules 1,850); Total fat 6g; Saturated fat 1g; Protein 11g; Cholesterol 4mg; Carbohydrates 88g; Sodium 595mg; Dietary fiber 3g; Calories from fat 12%

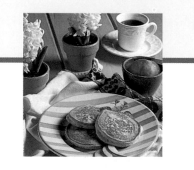

*Lemon-Poppy Seed Pancakes
with 2 tablespoons maple syrup*
page 64

1 nectarine

coffee or tea

Nutritional Analysis per Serving: Calories 468 (Kilojoules 1,965); Total fat 3g; Saturated fat 0g; Protein 11g; Cholesterol 1mg; Carbohydrates 102g; Sodium 482mg; Dietary fiber 4g; Calories from fat 5%

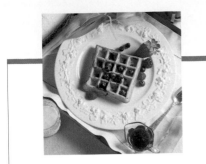

Very Berry Waffles
with 2 tablespoons maple syrup
page 67

Sunshine Smoothie
page 176

coffee or tea

Nutritional Analysis per Serving: Calories 554 (Kilojoules 2,325); Total fat 7g; Saturated fat 2g; Protein 12g; Cholesterol 6mg; Carbohydrates 115g; Sodium 649mg; Dietary fiber 7g; Calories from fat 11%

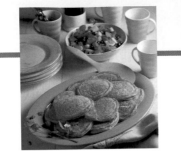

Multigrain Pancakes
page 68

Honey-Mint Fruit Compote
page 231

4 fl oz (125 ml) grapefruit juice

Nutritional Analysis per Serving: Calories 449 (Kilojoules 1,884); Total fat 6g; Saturated fat 1g; Protein 12g; Cholesterol 3mg; Carbohydrates 92g; Sodium 574mg; Dietary fiber 7g; Calories from fat 11%

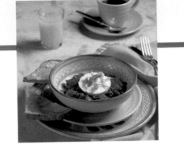

Santa Fe Eggs
page 71

1 slice multigrain toast
with 1 teaspoon margarine

4 fl oz (125 ml) orange juice

Nutritional Analysis per Serving: Calories 436 (Kilojoules 1,830); Total fat 13g; Saturated fat 3g; Protein 23g; Cholesterol 218mg; Carbohydrates 61g; Sodium 324mg; Dietary fiber 7g; Calories from fat 25%

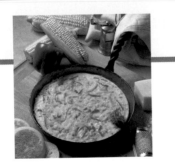

Green Pepper-Corn Frittata
page 72

½ toasted English muffin
with 2 teaspoons cream cheese

Strawberry-Banana Shake
page 176

Nutritional Analysis per Serving: Calories 383 (Kilojoules 1,609); Total fat 9g; Saturated fat 3g; Protein 14g; Cholesterol 118mg; Carbohydrates 65g; Sodium 700mg; Dietary fiber 6g; Calories from fat 21%

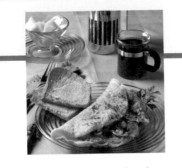

Onion-Mushroom Omelette
page 75

1 slice whole wheat toast
with 1 teaspoon margarine

¼ cantaloupe

coffee or tea

Nutritional Analysis per Serving: Calories 347 (Kilojoules 1,459); Total fat 11g; Saturated fat 2g; Protein 18g; Cholesterol 0mg; Carbohydrates 49g; Sodium 973mg; Dietary fiber 6g; Calories from fat 26%

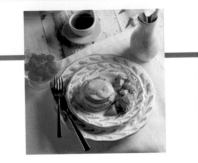

Eggs Benedict
with Lowfat Hollandaise
page 76

Rosemary Roasted Potatoes
page 202

1 cup (6 oz/185 g) watermelon
chunks

coffee or tea

Nutritional Analysis per Serving: Calories 492 (Kilojoules 2,067); Total fat 12g; Saturated fat 3g; Protein 22g; Cholesterol 274mg; Carbohydrates 74g; Sodium 752mg; Dietary fiber 5g; Calories from fat 23%

Poached Fruit with Cinnamon-Yogurt Topping

1½ cups (12 fl oz/375 ml)
  orange juice

¼ cup (2 fl oz/60 ml) water

1 tablespoon sugar

1 tablespoon raspberry or strawberry
  all-fruit preserves

2 teaspoons grated fresh ginger

4 whole cloves

1 vanilla bean (pod), 1½ inches
  (4 cm) long

2 oranges, peeled and sectioned

2 cups (8 oz/250 g) strawberries,
  stemmed and cored

Cinnamon-Yogurt Topping

1 cup (8 oz/250 g) nonfat
  plain yogurt

1 tablespoon sugar

1 teaspoon vanilla extract (essence)

1 teaspoon ground cinnamon

Shopping Tip

＊ All-fruit preserves are the type
sweetened with fruit juice rather
than added sugar.

Preparation: 15 minutes ＊ Cooking: 15 minutes ＊ Serves 4

Warm fruit with a dollop of spiced yogurt is the ideal comfort food to begin a chilly spring morning. Satisfying the requirement of 2 fruit servings for the entire day, it gets your healthy eating plan off to a good start.

＊ In a medium saucepan over high heat, combine the orange juice, water, sugar, preserves, ginger, cloves and vanilla bean. Bring to a boil, reduce the heat to low and simmer until the liquid thickens, about 10 minutes. Remove the vanilla bean, slice open and scrape out the seeds and return the seeds and split bean to the orange juice mixture.

＊ Add the orange sections and strawberries. Increase the heat to medium-high and return to a boil. Reduce the heat to medium-low and simmer until fruit is tender, about 2 minutes. Remove from the heat. Remove and discard the cloves and vanilla bean and seeds.

＊ To serve, divide the mixture among 4 individual bowls. Top each with an equal amount of the Cinnamon-Yogurt Topping.

Cinnamon-Yogurt Topping

＊ In a medium bowl, combine the yogurt, sugar, vanilla and cinnamon and whisk until blended.

Nutritional Analysis per Serving

Calories 157 (Kilojoules 660); Total fat 0g; Saturated fat 0g; Protein 5g; Cholesterol 1mg; Carbohydrates 35g; Sodium 45mg; Dietary fiber 3g; Calories from fat 2%

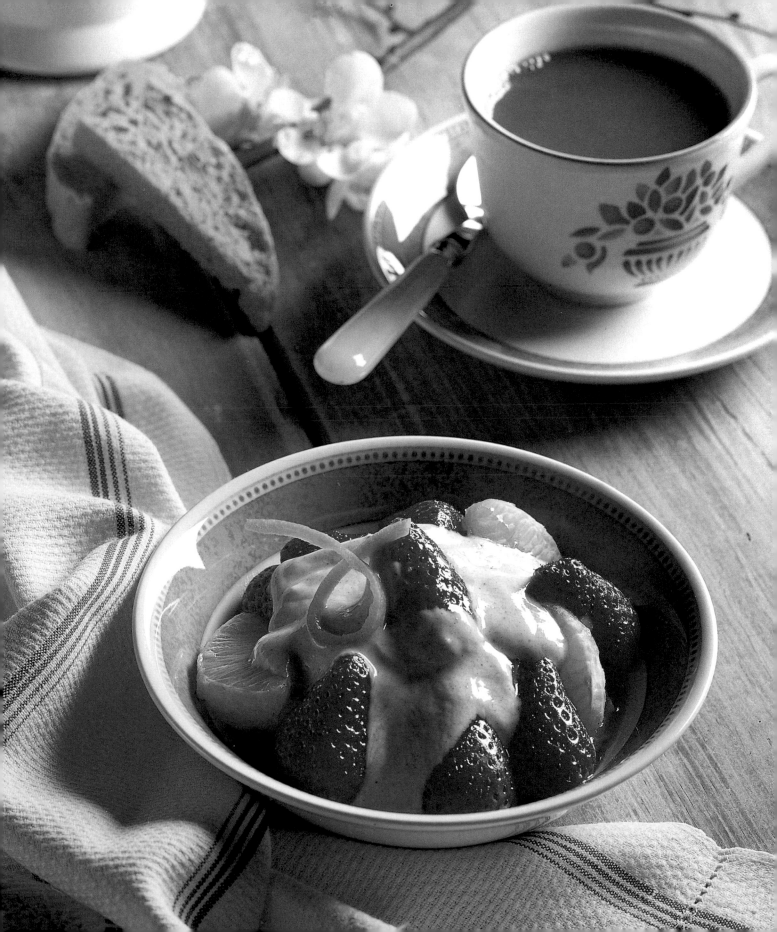

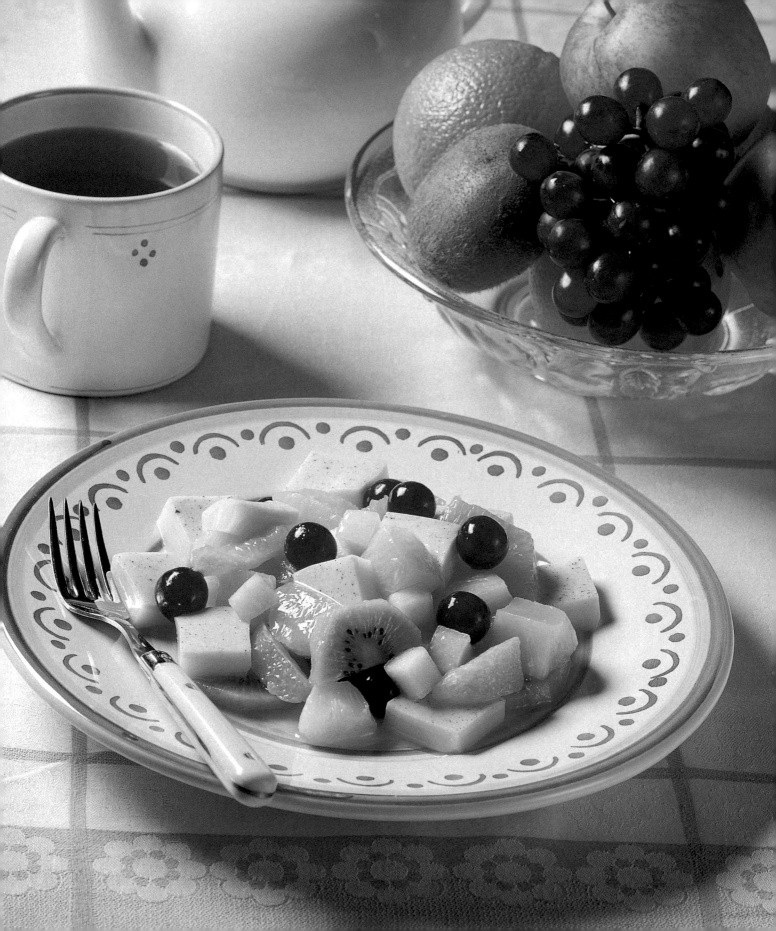

Almond Gelatin Squares in Fruit

Preparation: 15 minutes ✳ Chilling: 1 hour ✳ Serves 4

If you are short of time in the morning, make the gelatin the night before. The next morning, you'll need only a few minutes to toss the almond-laced gelatin squares with the mixed fruit.

4 teaspoons unflavored gelatin

½ cup (4 fl oz/125 ml) cold water

1½ cups (12 fl oz/375 ml) boiling water

¾ cup (3 oz/90 g) nonfat dry milk

½ cup (4 oz/125 g) sugar

1 teaspoon almond extract (essence)

¼ teaspoon ground cinnamon

1 pear, peeled, cored and cubed

1 cup (6 oz/185 g) seedless red grapes

2 kiwifruits, peeled and sliced

1 orange, peeled and sectioned

1⅓ cups (8 oz/250 g) pineapple chunks

¼ cup (2 fl oz/60 ml) orange juice

✳ In a small saucepan, combine the gelatin and cold water. Add the boiling water and stir until the gelatin is completely dissolved. Place over medium heat and bring to a boil, stirring constantly. Gradually whisk in the dry milk and sugar and return to a boil. Stir in the almond extract and cinnamon. When the cinnamon is dissolved, pour the mixture into an 8-inch (20-cm) square pan. Cover and refrigerate until firm, about 1 hour.

✳ In a large bowl, combine the pear, grapes, kiwifruits, orange, pineapple and orange juice. Gently toss to mix well.

✳ To serve, cut the gelatin into 1-inch (2.5-cm) squares, add to the fruit and toss gently. Divide among 4 individual bowls.

Nutrition Tip

✳ Kiwifruits, oranges and pineapples are all excellent sources of vitamin C.

Nutritional Analysis per Serving

Calories 323 (Kilojoules 1,356); Total fat 1g; Saturated fat 0g; Protein 11g; Cholesterol 4mg; Carbohydrates 71g; Sodium 125mg; Dietary fiber 5g; Calories from fat 2%

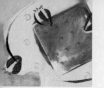

1 cup (4 oz/125 g) raspberries

1 cup (4 oz/125 g) blueberries

1 peach, pitted and sliced

1 pear, cored and sliced

1 cup (8 fl oz/250 ml) water

½ cup (4 fl oz/125 ml) apple juice

¼ cup (2 fl oz/60 ml) raspberry
    vinegar

¼ cup (2 oz/60 g) sugar

5 fresh rosemary sprigs

2 tablespoons finely grated
    lemon zest

Storage Tip

✴ If making the sauce ahead, store in an airtight container in the refrigerator and reheat in a small saucepan over low heat. The sauce is also delicious cold.

Summer Fruit in Rosemary Syrup

Preparation: 15 minutes ✶ *Cooking: 15 minutes* ✶ *Serves 4*

Rosemary, the symbolic herb of remembrance, lends its pungent flavor and aroma to this colorful fruit mix. Both the leaves and the pale purple flowers are edible. Be sure to crush the needlelike leaves to release their oils as you add the herb to the saucepan.

✶ Divide the raspberries, blueberries, peach slices and pear slices among 4 individual bowls.

✶ To make the rosemary syrup, in a small saucepan over medium-high heat, combine the water, apple juice, vinegar, sugar, rosemary and lemon zest. Bring to a boil, reduce the heat to low and simmer until the liquid is reduced by half, about 10 minutes. Cool for 5 minutes. Strain the syrup through a fine-mesh sieve.

✶ To serve, pour an equal amount of the rosemary syrup over each bowl of fruit.

Nutritional Analysis per Serving

Calories 142 (Kilojoules 598); Total fat 1g; Saturated fat 0g; Protein 1g; Cholesterol 0mg; Carbohydrates 36g; Sodium 3mg; Dietary fiber 4g; Calories from fat 3%

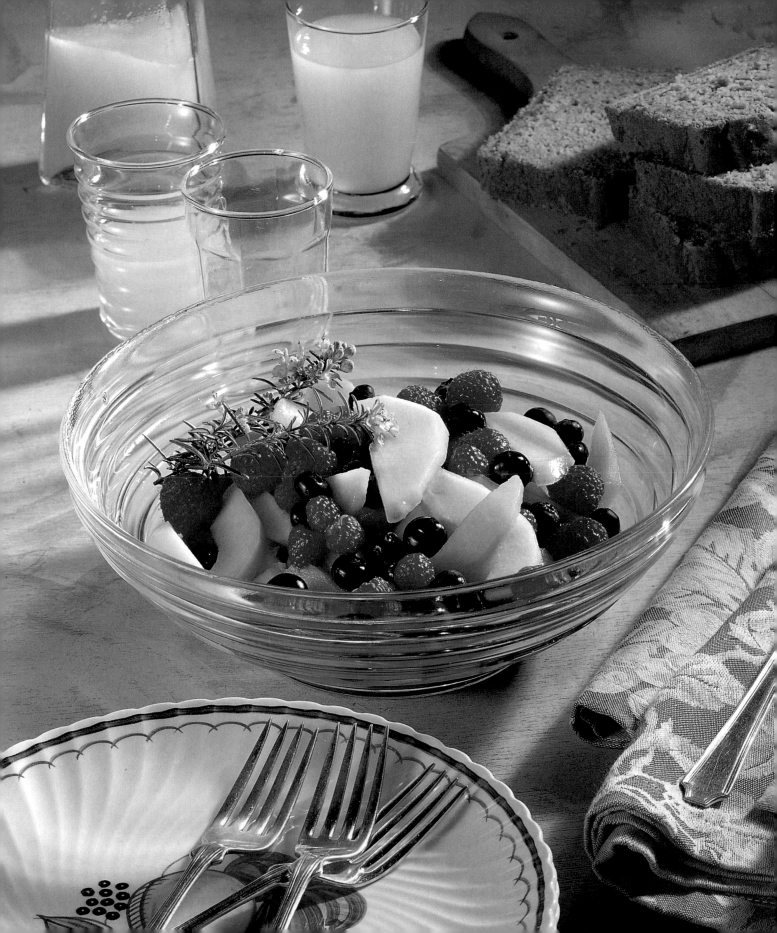

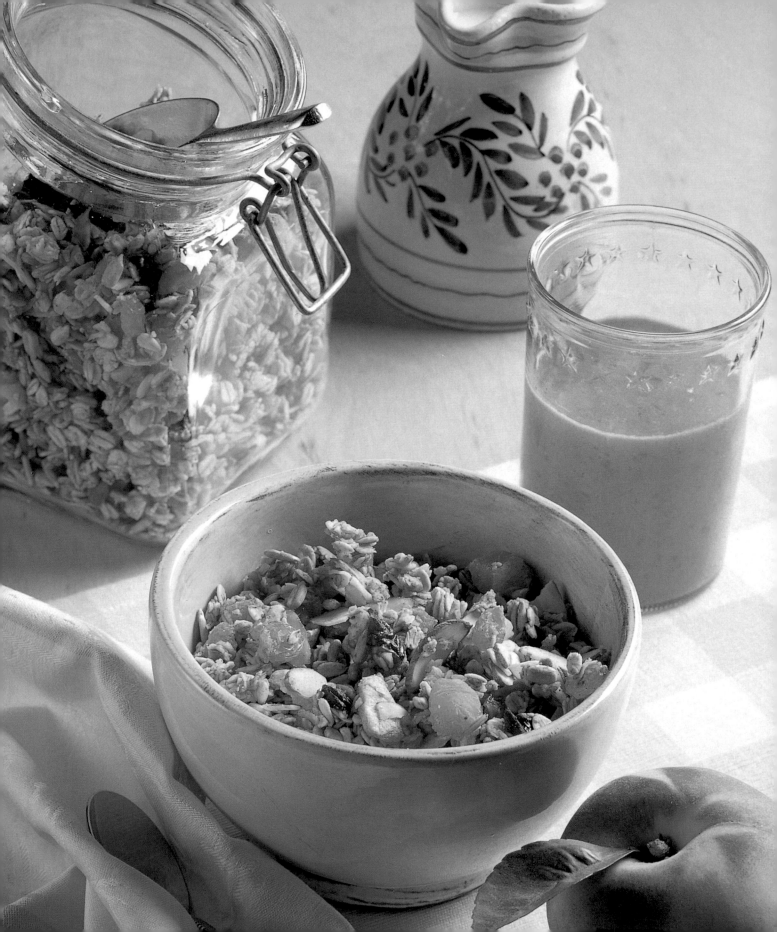

Hearty Granola

½ cup (3 oz/90 g) raisins

¼ cup (2 oz/60 g) chopped dried prunes

¼ cup (2 oz/60 g) chopped dried apples

¼ cup (2 oz/60 g) chopped dried apricots

1 cup (8 fl oz/250 ml) hot water

3 cups (9 oz/280 g) rolled oats

1½ cups (4½ oz/140 g) unsweetened puffed rice cereal

½ cup (2 oz/60 g) raw sunflower seeds

½ cup (2 oz/60 g) sliced (flaked) almonds

¼ cup (1 oz/30 g) nonfat dry milk

2 tablespoons shredded unsweetened coconut

2 tablespoons honey

1 teaspoon ground cinnamon

*Preparation: 25 minutes * Cooking: 1 hour * Makes 7 cups*

Ted is a big granola fan and really likes this version. It's great with milk as a breakfast cereal, plain as a snack or sprinkled over yogurt as a dessert. Consider making several batches and filling decorative airtight jars to give as gifts. Include a copy of the nutritional analysis and inspire others to take the road to healthy eating.

✳ Preheat an oven to 250°F (120°C).

✳ In a small bowl, soak the raisins and dried fruit in the hot water until softened, 15 minutes. In a large bowl, combine the oats, rice cereal, sunflower seeds, almonds, dry milk, coconut, honey and cinnamon. Add the raisins and fruit with the soaking water. Stir to mix well.

✳ Spread the mixture on a baking sheet and bake for 1 hour, stirring every 15 minutes to prevent sticking and to ensure even cooking. Remove from the oven and cool. One serving is 1 cup (6 oz/180 g).

✳ To store, place in an airtight container for up to 1 week.

Nutritional Analysis per Serving

Calories 443 (Kilojoules 1,861); Total fat 12g; Saturated fat 2g; Protein 13g; Cholesterol 1mg; Carbohydrates 77g; Sodium 36mg; Dietary fiber 6g; Calories from fat 22%

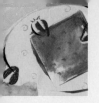

2½ cups (20 fl oz/625 ml) apple cider
    or apple juice
¼ cup (1½ oz/45 g) raisins
1 apple, peeled, cored and diced
¾ teaspoon ground cinnamon
1½ cups (4½ oz/140 g) rolled oats
½ cup (4 oz/125 g) nonfat
    plain yogurt
1 teaspoon ground nutmeg

Apple-Raisin Oatmeal

Preparation: 10 minutes ✳ Cooking: 10 minutes ✳ Serves 4

When I was about 10 years old, I had an exam at school that was very important. That morning I ate a big bowl of hot oatmeal, something I was not accustomed to doing. I did great on the exam and began calling oatmeal "brain food." Now I know that my childhood instincts were remarkably accurate. A hearty breakfast of complex carbohydrates like those found in oatmeal increases your attention span and ability to concentrate. I still eat it whenever I have something important to do.

✳ In a medium saucepan over medium-high heat, bring the cider or juice to a boil. Stir in the raisins, apple and cinnamon, reduce the heat to low and simmer for 2 minutes. Stir in the oats, increase the heat to medium-high and bring to a boil. Reduce the heat to low and simmer, stirring frequently, until the liquid is absorbed and the oats are creamy, about 6 minutes.

✳ To serve, divide among 4 individual bowls. Top each with an equal amount of the yogurt and nutmeg.

Nutritional Analysis per Serving

Calories 265 (Kilojoules 1,115); Total fat 3g; Saturated fat 1g; Protein 7g;
Cholesterol 1mg; Carbohydrates 55g; Sodium 29mg; Dietary fiber 4g;
Calories from fat 8%

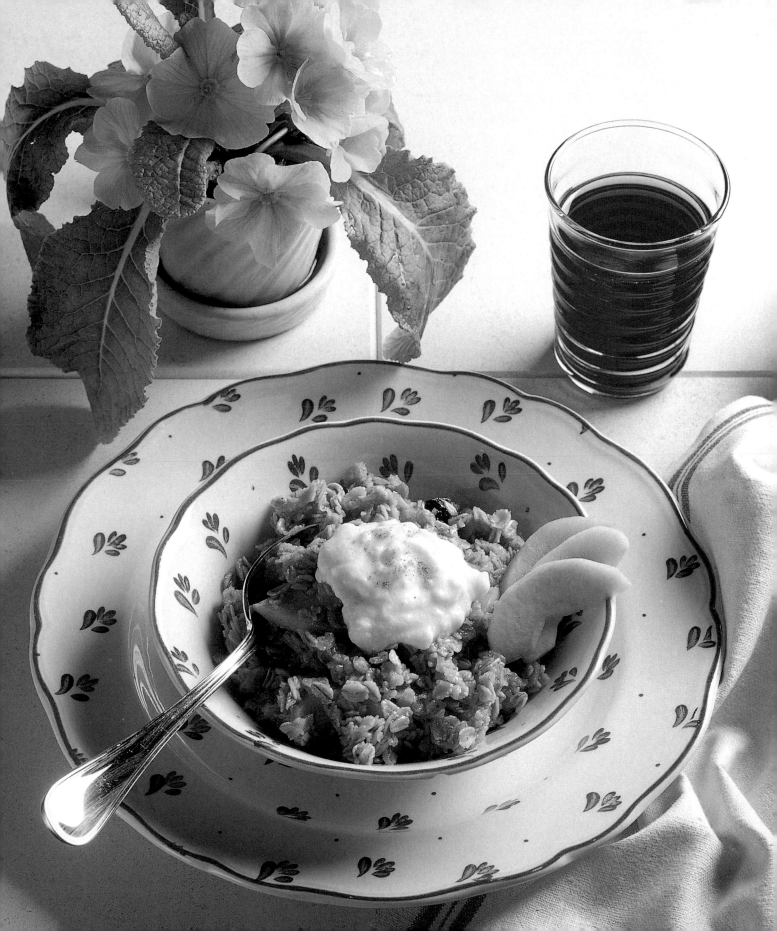

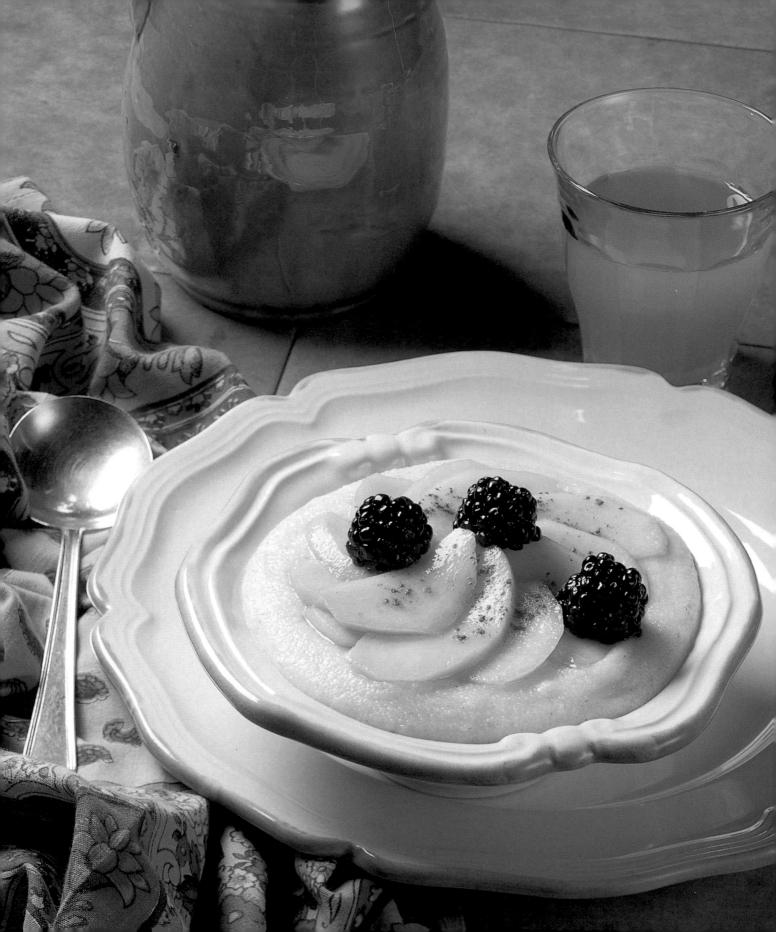

Hot Wheat Cereal with Gingered Peaches

Preparation: 5 minutes ✳ Cooking: 15 minutes ✳ Serves 4

Notice that this creamy white cereal with warm fruit has no cholesterol and derives just 2 percent of its calories from fat. It makes a good alternative to oatmeal for a hot breakfast cereal and provides a grain and a fruit serving, essential components of your daily food needs.

4½ cups (36 fl oz/1.12 l) water

¾ cup (6 oz/185 g) enriched farina wheat cereal

1½ cups (12 fl oz/375 ml) apple juice

1 tablespoon grated fresh ginger

4 peaches, peeled, pitted and sliced

¼ cup (2 fl oz/60 ml) raspberry vinegar

3 tablespoons honey

½ teaspoon ground cinnamon

12 blackberries

✳ In a medium saucepan over medium-high heat, bring the water to a boil. Stir in the wheat cereal, reduce the heat to low and simmer, stirring frequently, until thickened, about 10 minutes.

✳ To make the gingered peaches, in a small saucepan over high heat, combine the apple juice, ginger and peaches. Bring to a boil, reduce the heat to low and simmer until the liquid is reduced by half, about 10 minutes. Add the vinegar, honey and cinnamon. Increase the heat to medium-high, bring to a boil, reduce the heat to low and simmer until the peaches are tender, about 5 minutes.

✳ To serve, divide the cereal among 4 individual bowls. Top each with an equal amount of the gingered peaches and blackberries.

Nutritional Analysis per Serving

Calories 309 (Kilojoules 1,300); Total fat 1g; Saturated fat 0g; Protein 5g; Cholesterol 0mg; Carbohydrates 72g; Sodium 7mg; Dietary fiber 4g; Calories from fat 2%

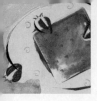

4 cups (32 fl oz/1 l) water

1 teaspoon salt

1 cup (6 oz/185 g) steel-cut oats

4 teaspoons brown sugar

Nutrition Tip

✳ Try gradually decreasing the amount of salt each time you make oatmeal. The oat flavor is rich and full without a lot of added sodium.

Irish Oatmeal

Preparation: 5 minutes ✳ *Cooking: 30 minutes* ✳ *Serves 4*

Karen Averitt serves this nearly every morning at our Montana ranch. It offers a great start to our busy days filled with outdoor activities. Also known as Irish oats, steel-cut oats need to cook longer than rolled oats, but have a wonderfully hearty, chewy texture.

✳ In a medium saucepan over medium-high heat, combine the water and salt. Bring to a boil. Gradually add the oats, stirring constantly. Reduce the heat to low and simmer, stirring frequently, until the water is absorbed and the oats are creamy, about 30 minutes.

✳ To serve, divide among 4 individual bowls. Top each with an equal amount of the brown sugar.

Nutritional Analysis per Serving

Calories 181 (Kilojoules 758); Total fat 3g; Saturated fat 0g; Protein 7g; Cholesterol 0mg; Carbohydrates 33g; Sodium 554mg; Dietary fiber 4g; Calories from fat 13%

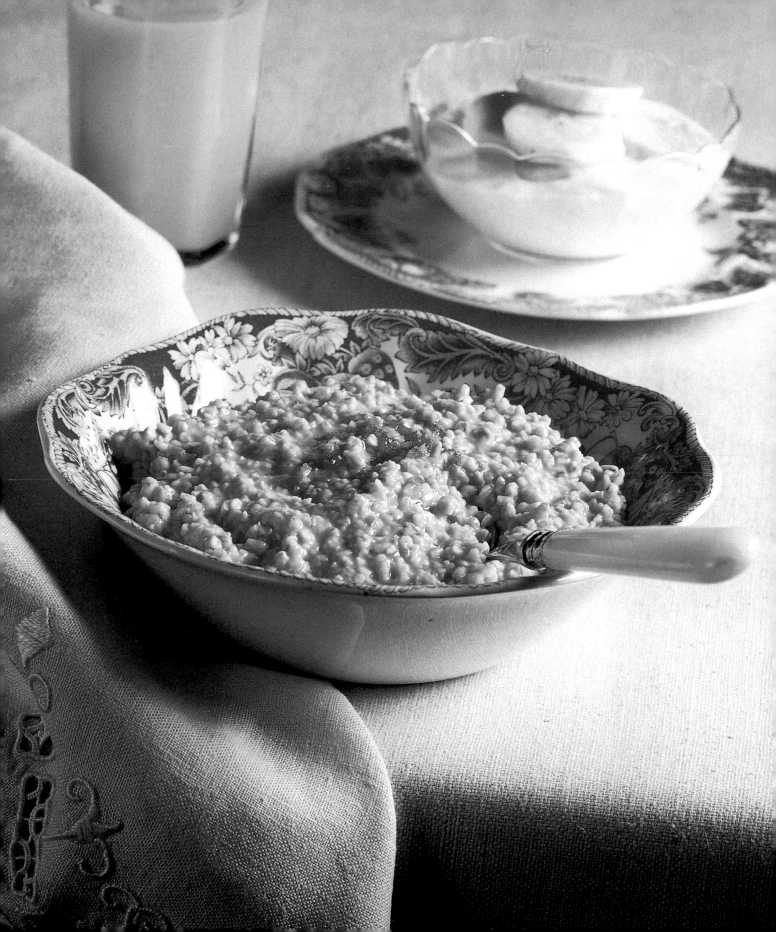

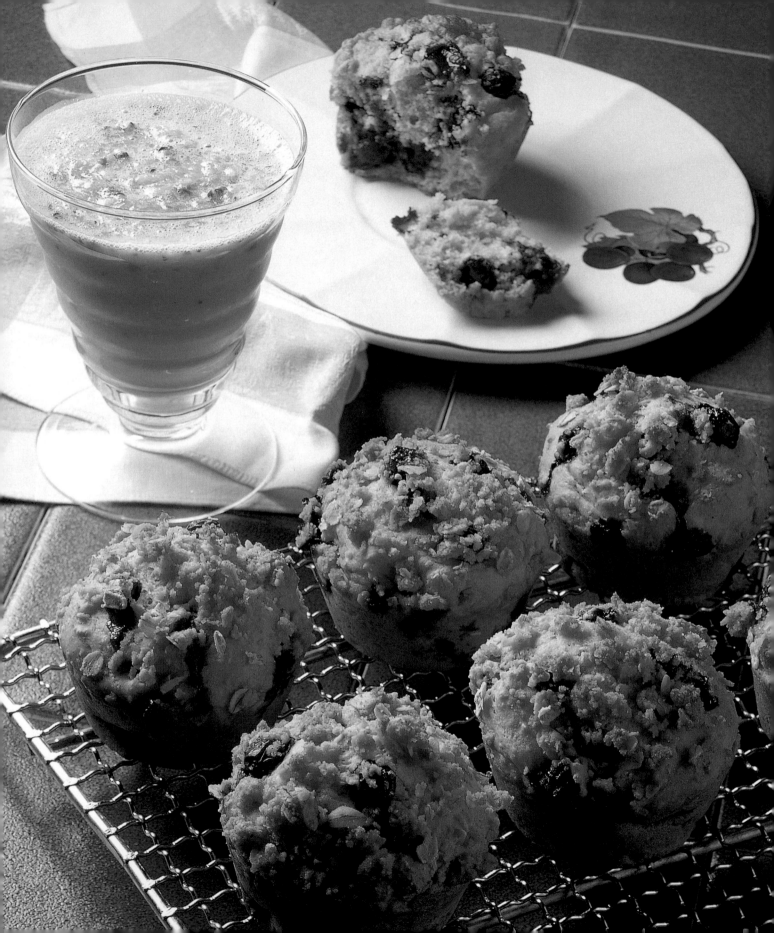

Blueberry Muffins

Preparation: 25 minutes ✳ *Cooking: 20 minutes* ✳ *Serves 18*

The crunchy topping adds texture—and extra fiber—to these muffins. The recipe makes enough for several breakfasts and healthy midday snacks.

✳ Preheat an oven to 400°F (200°C). Coat tins for 18 muffins with nonstick cooking spray (or line with paper muffin cups).

✳ In a large bowl, combine the 2 cups unbleached flour, whole wheat flour, ½ cup brown sugar, baking powder, baking soda, salt and lemon zest. Make a well in the center of the dry ingredients. In a medium bowl, whisk together the buttermilk, oil and vanilla. Pour the buttermilk mixture into the well in the dry ingredients and stir until just blended. Fold in the blueberries. Spoon the batter into the prepared muffin tins.

✳ To make the topping, in a small bowl, combine the oats, 3 tablespoons flour, 3 tablespoons brown sugar and margarine and stir to blend. Sprinkle an equal amount of topping over each muffin.

✳ Bake the muffins until golden brown and a toothpick inserted in the center of a middle muffin comes out clean, about 20 minutes. Cool for 10 minutes.

✳ To serve, arrange on a serving plate. One serving is 1 muffin. Store wrapped individually in plastic wrap in an airtight container in the freezer for up to 3 months.

---

2 cups (10 oz/315 g) plus 3 tablespoons unbleached flour

1½ cups (7½ oz/235 g) whole wheat (wholemeal) flour

½ cup (3½ oz/105 g) plus 3 tablespoons brown sugar

1 tablespoon baking powder

1½ teaspoons baking soda (bicarbonate of soda)

½ teaspoon salt

1 teaspoon finely grated lemon zest

2⅓ cups (19 fl oz/580 ml) lowfat buttermilk

1 tablespoon vegetable oil

1½ teaspoons vanilla extract (essence)

2 cups (8 oz/250 g) blueberries

3 tablespoons quick-cooking oats

1½ tablespoons margarine

Shopping Tip

✳ Look for fresh blueberries at the height of summer. Chose firm, plump berries and remove any stems before use. Large berries have more flavor than small ones. If using frozen or canned blueberries, seek brands packed in water rather than a sugary syrup, and drain and blot off all excess liquid.

Nutritional Analysis per Serving

Calories 172 (Kilojoules 724); Total fat 3g; Saturated fat 0g; Protein 5g; Cholesterol 1mg; Carbohydrates 33g; Sodium 296mg; Dietary fiber 2g; Calories from fat 13%

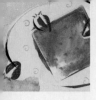

Banana Bread

Preparation: 20 minutes ✳ *Cooking: 1 hour* ✳ *Serves 8*

The perfect solution for using bananas that are too ripe to eat out of hand is to make banana bread. Bananas are high in potassium, niacin and vitamins A and C.

✳ Preheat an oven to 350°F (180°C). Coat a 9-by-5-inch (23-by-13-cm) loaf pan with nonstick cooking spray.

✳ In a large bowl, combine the flour, baking powder, baking soda and salt. Make a well in the center of the dry ingredients. In a medium bowl, mash the bananas until smooth. Add the egg whites, sugar, buttermilk and vanilla and stir to mix well. Pour the banana mixture into the well in the dry ingredients and fold together until blended.

✳ Pour the batter into the prepared loaf pan and bake until a toothpick inserted in the center comes out clean, 55–60 minutes. Cool for 10 minutes.

✳ To serve, cut into 8 slices. One serving is 1 slice. Store wrapped in plastic wrap in an airtight container in the freezer for up to 1 month.

2 cups (10 oz/315 g) unbleached flour

2 teaspoons baking powder

½ teaspoon baking soda (bicarbonate of soda)

½ teaspoon salt

4 large, overripe bananas

2 egg whites

¾ cup (6 oz/185 g) sugar

¼ cup (2 fl oz/60 ml) lowfat buttermilk

1 teaspoon vanilla extract (essence)

Shopping Tip

✳ Bananas are grown in South and Central America and are shipped throughout the world. Often picked while still green, they continue to ripen after harvesting. Purchase plump specimens with unblemished skins. Stored at room temperature, the fruit will ripen in 2 to 3 days. Ripe bananas are uniformly yellow, speckled with brown spots. They need to be very ripe for use in bread.

Nutritional Analysis per Serving

Calories 282 (Kilojoules 1,183); Total fat 1g; Saturated fat 0g; Protein 5g; Cholesterol 0mg; Carbohydrates 64g; Sodium 360mg; Dietary fiber 2g; Calories from fat 3%

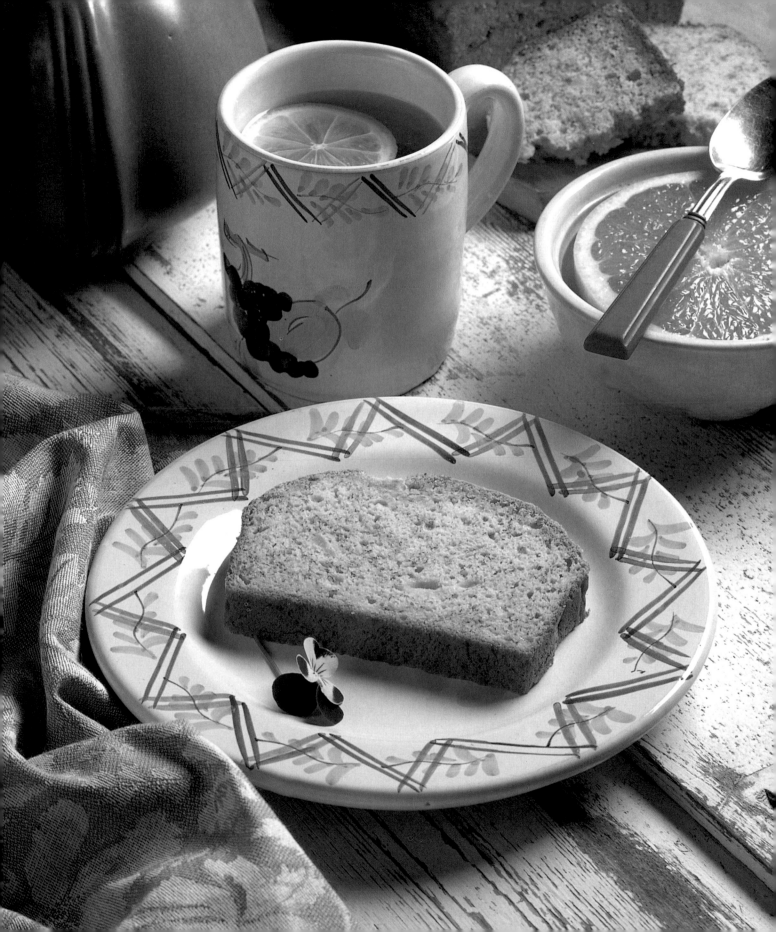

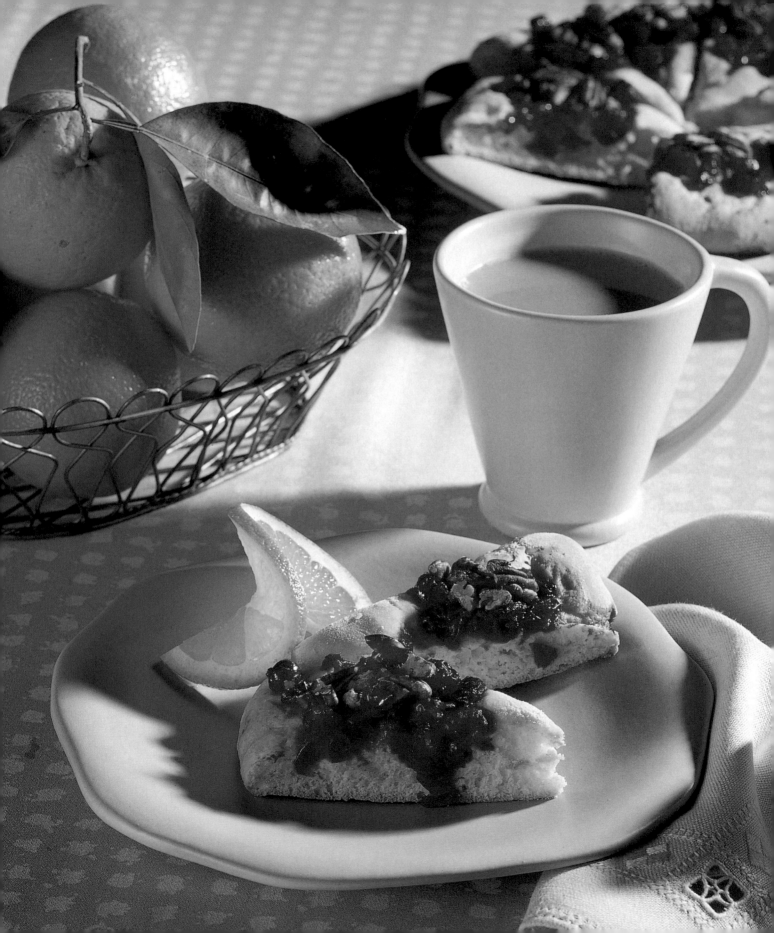

Cranberry-Pecan Scones

1½ cups (6 oz/185 g) fresh cranberries

2 tablespoons water

½ cup (4 oz/120 g) sugar

1 tablespoon brown sugar

2 cups (10 oz/315 g) unbleached flour

2 teaspoons baking powder

½ teaspoon baking soda
(bicarbonate of soda)

¼ teaspoon salt

2 tablespoons margarine cut into
small pieces

¾ cup (6 fl oz/180 ml) lowfat
buttermilk

1 egg white

¼ cup (1 oz/30 g) chopped pecans

Preparation: 20 minutes ✳ *Cooking: 25 minutes* ✳ *Serves 6*

Cranberries, the fruit of a low-lying vine native to North America, are a good source of vitamin C and high in fiber. Wild versions were an important nutrient for Native Americans.

✳ Preheat an oven to 400°F (200°C). Coat a baking sheet with nonstick cooking spray.

✳ In a small saucepan over medium heat, combine the cranberries, water and half the sugar. Simmer until the cranberries are tender and the mixture thickens, about 10 minutes.

✳ In a food processor with the metal blade or by hand in a large bowl, combine the remaining sugar, brown sugar, flour, baking powder, baking soda and salt. Process or stir to mix well. Add the margarine and process or use a fork to blend until the mixture resembles coarse meal.

✳ In a small bowl, combine the buttermilk and egg white. Stir into the flour mixture.

✳ Turn the dough onto a lightly floured work surface and knead gently about 5 times. Form into a ball, place on the prepared baking sheet and press into an 8-inch (20-cm) round. Using a lightly floured knife, cut the round into 12 wedges without cutting completely through to the baking sheet. Spoon an equal amount of the cranberry mixture onto the center of each wedge and press down gently with the back of the spoon. Top with an equal amount of the pecans. Bake until golden brown and a toothpick inserted in the center comes out clean, 13–15 minutes. Cool for 10 minutes.

✳ To serve, cut into 12 pieces. One serving is 2 scones. Store wrapped in plastic wrap in the refrigerator for up to 3 days.

Shopping Tip

✳ Fresh cranberries are available in the fall. During other times of the year, substitute frozen, whole, unsweetened cranberries or dried cranberries.

Nutritional Analysis per Serving

Calories 350 (Kilojoules 1,470); Total fat 8g; Saturated fat 1g; Protein 7g; Cholesterol 1mg; Carbohydrates 64g; Sodium 445mg; Dietary fiber 3g; Calories from fat 20%

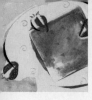

2 cups (8 oz/250 g) grated, packed
   tart apples (about 3)
2 tablespoons lemon juice
½ teaspoon finely grated lemon zest
¼ cup (2 oz/60 g) light brown sugar
¼ cup (3 oz/90 g) honey
2 tablespoons margarine, melted
2 tablespoons nonfat milk
1 egg
2 cups (10 oz/315 g) unbleached flour
2 teaspoons baking powder
½ teaspoon baking soda
   (bicarbonate of soda)
1¼ teaspoons ground cinnamon
¼ teaspoon salt
⅓ cup (1¼ oz/40 g) chopped walnuts

Cooking Tip

✳ For a heartier texture, dice the apples instead of grating them. For an aromatic change of pace, add ¼ teaspoon of ground allspice, nutmeg or ginger along with the cinnamon.

Apple-Walnut Bread

Preparation: 20 minutes ✳ Cooking: 1 hour ✳ Serves 8

Tart apples, including Granny Smiths, pippins and Gravensteins, work best for baking. Save sweeter apples such as Red and Golden Delicious, McIntosh and Winesap for eating out of hand. All apples are high in fiber, water and pectin, which helps lower cholesterol levels, and are a good source of vitamin C.

✳ Preheat an oven to 350°F (180°C). Coat a 9-by-5-inch (23-by-13-cm) loaf pan with nonstick cooking spray.

✳ In a medium bowl, combine the apples, lemon juice and lemon zest. Stir to mix well. In a large bowl, whisk together the brown sugar, honey, margarine, milk and egg. Stir in the apple mixture. In another large bowl, sift together the flour, baking powder, baking soda, cinnamon and salt. Make a well in the center of the dry ingredients. Pour the apple mixture into the well and fold together until blended. Fold in the walnuts.

✳ Pour the batter into the prepared loaf pan and bake until a toothpick inserted in the center comes out clean, about 1 hour. If it begins to over-brown during cooking, cover the top of the bread with foil. Cool for 10 minutes.

✳ To serve, cut into 8 slices. One serving is 1 slice. Store in an airtight container in the freezer for up to 3 months.

Nutritional Analysis per Serving

Calories 272 (Kilojoules 1,144); Total fat 7g; Saturated fat 1g; Protein 5g; Cholesterol 27mg; Carbohydrates 49g; Sodium 316mg; Dietary fiber 2g; Calories from fat 22%

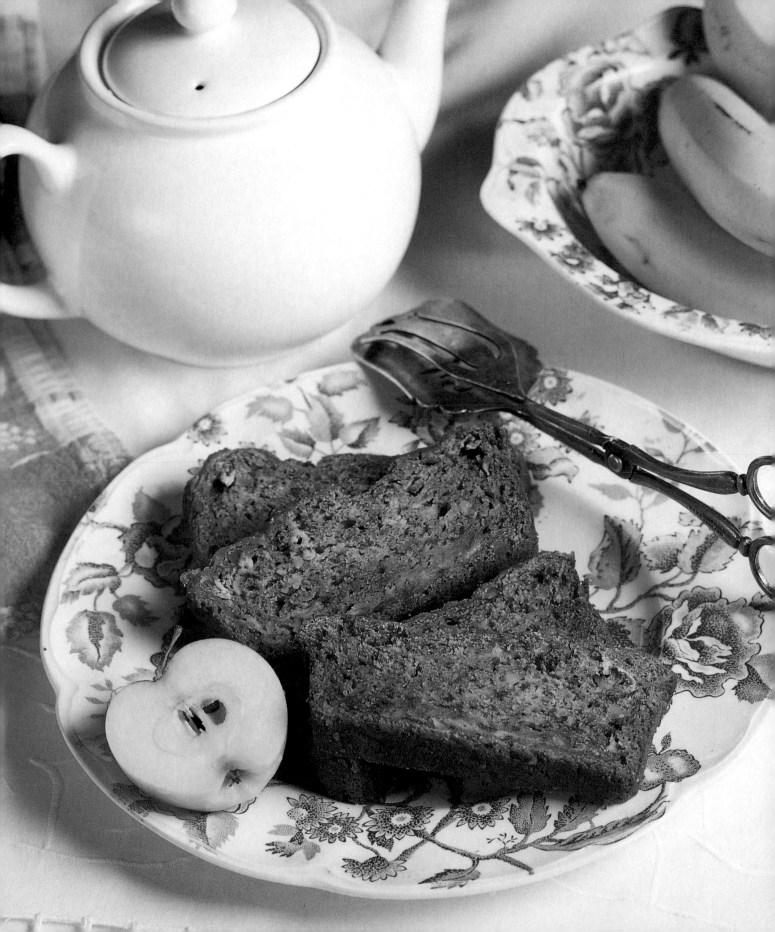

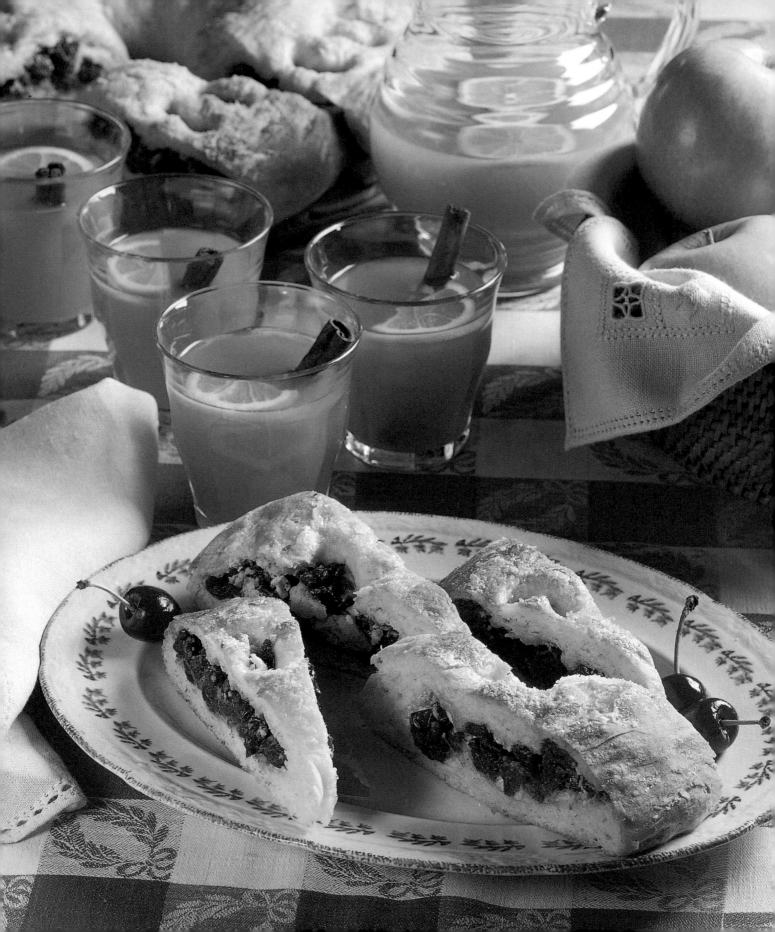

2 teaspoons active dry yeast

1¼ cups (10 fl oz/310 ml) warm water

½ tablespoon margarine, melted

5 tablespoons sugar

½ teaspoon salt

3½ cups (17½ oz/545 g) unbleached
   flour

1½ lb (750 g) cherries, pitted

8 oz (250 g) nonfat cream cheese

¼ cup (2 oz/60 g) nonfat plain yogurt

½ teaspoon vanilla extract (essence)

1 tablespoon nonfat milk

Shopping Tip

✻ In winter, substitute 32 oz (1 kg)
canned pitted sour cherries in water for
the fresh cherries. To shorten preparation
time, use thawed frozen Italian bread
dough in place of this homemade version.

Cherry-Cheese Coffee Ring

Preparation: 20 minutes ✻ Cooking: 45 minutes ✻ Serves 8

*In addition to the preparation and cooking times noted above, this dough
needs to rise for 1 hour and 45 minutes before baking.*

✻ In a large bowl, dissolve the yeast in the water and let stand for
5 minutes. Add the margarine, 3 tablespoons of the sugar, the salt
and flour and work into a dough. Using a mixer with a dough
hook or by hand on a lightly floured work surface, knead the
dough until smooth and elastic, about 4 minutes. Form into a
ball. Coat a large bowl with nonstick cooking spray, add the dough
and turn to coat all sides. Cover with a kitchen towel and let
rise in a warm place, free from draft, until doubled, about 1 hour.

✻ In a medium saucepan over medium heat, place the cherries
in water to cover and bring to a boil. Reduce the heat to low
and simmer for 10 minutes. Drain well, blot to remove all excess
liquid and cool.

✻ In a food processor with the metal blade or in a blender, combine the cream cheese, yogurt and vanilla and process until smooth.

✻ Punch down the dough and roll out to an 8-by-14-inch (20-
by-35-cm) rectangle. Spread the cream cheese mixture over the
dough to within 1 inch (2.5 cm) of the edges. Top with the
cherries. Fold the dough over lengthwise and pinch the edges
to seal. Coat a baking sheet with nonstick cooking spray. On the
baking sheet, form the dough into a ring. Using kitchen scissors,
make deep cuts all around the top of the ring. Cover with a
kitchen towel and let rise until doubled in bulk, about 45 minutes.

✻ Preheat an oven to 375°F (190°C). Brush the top of the ring
with the milk and sprinkle with the remaining sugar. Bake until
golden brown, about 30 minutes. Cool for 10 minutes.

✻ To serve, cut into 8 pieces. One serving is 1 piece.

Nutritional Analysis per Serving

Calories 334 (Kilojoules 1,401); Total fat 2g; Saturated fat 0g; Protein 12g;
Cholesterol 3mg; Carbohydrates 67g; Sodium 291mg; Dietary fiber 2g;
Calories from fat 5%

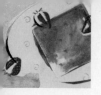

1 cup (8 oz/250 g) plus 2 tablespoons
  sugar

½ cup (3½ oz/105 g) brown sugar

8 oz (250 g) nonfat cream cheese

2 tablespoons margarine

3 egg whites

1 teaspoon vanilla extract (essence)

2 cups (10 oz/315 g) unbleached flour

2 teaspoons baking powder

¼ teaspoon ground nutmeg

¼ teaspoon salt

2 cups (8 oz/250 g) blueberries

1 teaspoon ground cinnamon

Cooking Tip

* Folding is a slightly different technique than simply stirring ingredients to combine them. The purpose of folding a batter is to add air while incorporating a heavier ingredient into a lighter one. When folding the blueberries into this coffee cake batter, for example, use a rubber spatula to cut repeatedly through the batter in a down, across and upward motion.

Blueberry Coffee Cake

Preparation: 20 minutes ✴ *Cooking: 35 minutes* ✴ *Serves 8*

Using egg whites only, rather than the whole eggs, lowers the fat and cholesterol in this coffee cake without sacrificing any of the flavor.

✴ Preheat an oven to 350°F (180°C). Coat a bundt pan or 9-by-13-inch (23-by-33-cm) baking pan with nonstick cooking spray.

✴ To make the cake, in a large bowl using an electric mixer or by hand, beat the 1 cup sugar, brown sugar, cream cheese and margarine until creamy. Add the egg whites and vanilla and beat until smooth. In a small bowl, combine the flour, baking powder, nutmeg and salt. Stir the flour mixture into the cream cheese mixture. Fold in the blueberries. Pour the batter into the prepared pan.

✴ To make the topping, in a small bowl, combine the 2 tablespoons sugar and cinnamon and sprinkle over the batter.

✴ Bake until a toothpick inserted in the center comes out clean, about 1 hour in a bundt pan and about 35 minutes in a baking pan. Cool for 10 minutes.

✴ To serve, cut into 8 pieces. One serving is 1 piece. Store wrapped in plastic wrap in the refrigerator for up to 3 days.

Nutritional Analysis per Serving

Calories 374 (Kilojoules 1,573); Total fat 3g; Saturated fat 1g; Protein 9g; Cholesterol 3mg; Carbohydrates 77g; Sodium 386mg; Dietary fiber 2g; Calories from fat 8%

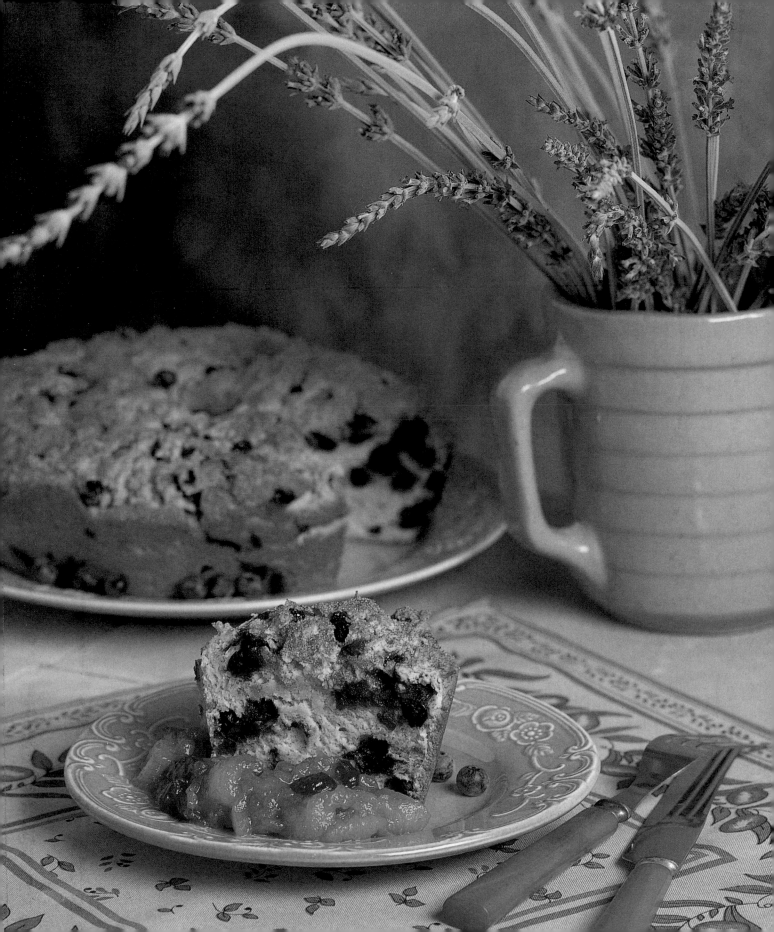

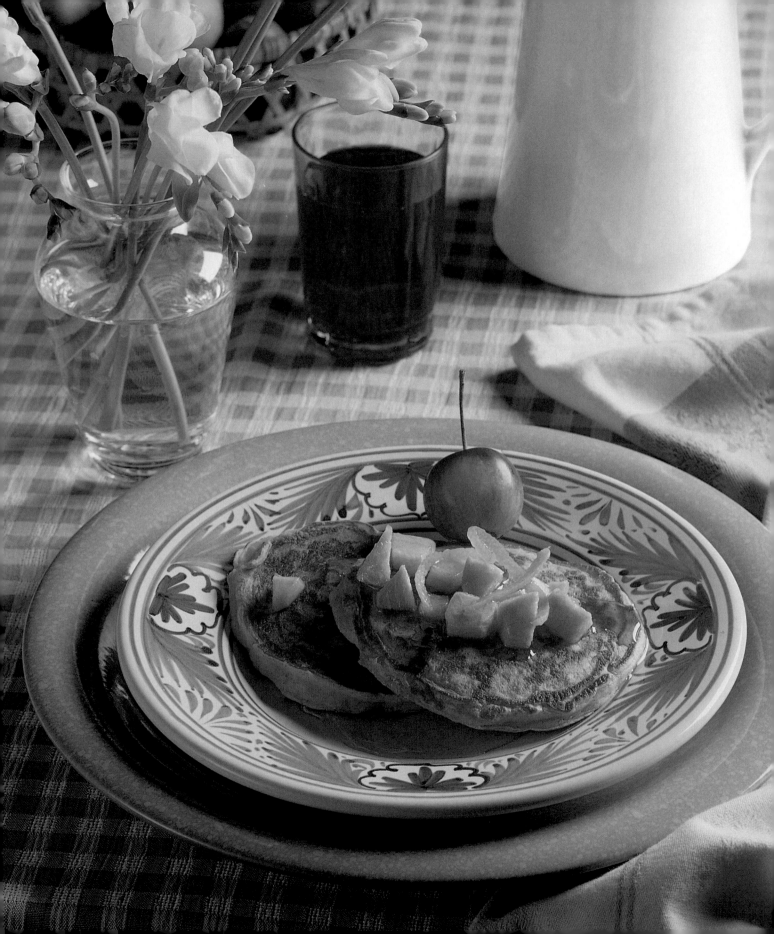

Oat-Buttermilk Pancakes with Honey-Fruit Sauce

1½ cups (12 fl oz/375 ml) lowfat
   buttermilk

¾ cup (2¼ oz/65 g) rolled oats

1 tablespoon margarine, melted

2 egg whites

½ teaspoon vanilla extract (essence)

1 cup (5 oz/155 g) unbleached flour

2 tablespoons brown sugar

½ teaspoon baking soda
   (bicarbonate of soda)

½ teaspoon salt

¼ teaspoon ground nutmeg

Honey-Fruit Sauce

1 pear, peeled, cored and diced

1 tart apple, peeled, cored and diced

1 cup (12 oz/375 g) honey

1 tablespoon lemon juice

1 teaspoon finely grated lemon zest

¼ teaspoon ground cinnamon

4 whole cloves

Cooking Tip

✳ Pancakes have the best texture when the batter is made just before cooking because any storage time causes the baking soda to lose its punch.

Preparation: 15 minutes ✳ Cooking: 10 minutes ✳ Serves 4

Rolled oats add texture and fiber to old-fashioned buttermilk pancakes. Prepare the sauce before the pancakes.

✳ In a large bowl, combine the buttermilk, oats, margarine, egg whites and vanilla. Let stand for 10 minutes. In a large bowl, combine the flour, brown sugar, baking soda, salt and nutmeg. Add the flour mixture to the buttermilk mixture and stir to mix well.

✳ Coat a griddle or large nonstick frying pan with nonstick cooking spray. Place over medium–high heat until hot. The griddle is the right temperature when water dropped on the surface bounces and dances. If the water evaporates immediately, the griddle is too hot; if the water sits still, the griddle is not hot enough. Spoon the batter in scant ⅓-cup (2½-oz/75-g) portions onto the hot griddle to make 12 pancakes. Flip each pancake when the surface is covered with tiny bubbles, about 3 minutes. Cook until the bottom is golden brown, about 2 minutes more.

✳ To serve, divide among 4 individual plates. One serving is 3 pancakes.

Honey-Fruit Sauce

✳ In a small saucepan over medium heat, combine the pear, apple, honey, lemon juice, lemon zest, cinnamon and cloves. Bring to a boil, reduce the heat to low and simmer until the fruit is tender, about 5 minutes. Remove and discard the cloves.

✳ To serve, spoon the hot sauce over the pancakes. One serving is 2 tablespoons. Store in an airtight container in the refrigerator for up to 1 week. Reheat before serving.

Nutritional Analysis per Serving

Calories 368 (Kilojoules 1,547); Total fat 6g; Saturated fat 1g; Protein 11g; Cholesterol 4mg; Carbohydrates 70g; Sodium 592mg; Dietary fiber 3g; Calories from fat 13%

Lemon-Poppy Seed Pancakes

1½ cups (7½ oz/235 g)
   unbleached flour

¼ cup (2 oz/60 g) sugar

1 tablespoon poppy seeds

1 teaspoon baking powder

½ teaspoon baking soda
   (bicarbonate of soda)

¼ teaspoon salt

¾ cup (6 fl oz/180 ml) nonfat milk

¼ cup (2 oz/60 g) nonfat plain yogurt

2 egg whites

1 tablespoon lemon juice

2 teaspoons finely grated lemon zest

Storage Tip

✳ Poppy seeds contain a lot of oil and
go rancid quickly. Store in an airtight
container in a cool, dark place for up
to 6 months.

Preparation: 15 minutes ✳ Cooking: 10 minutes ✳ Serves 4

*Several types of poppy plants provide edible seeds. Some seeds are white;
most are black. Both have a slightly sweet, nutty flavor. If desired, lightly
toast the seeds before using to bring out more of their distinctive flavor.*

✳ In a large bowl, combine the flour, sugar, poppy seeds, baking
powder, baking soda and salt. Make a well in the center. In another
large bowl, whisk together the milk, yogurt, egg whites, lemon
juice and lemon zest. Pour the milk mixture into the well in the
flour mixture and stir to mix well.

✳ Coat a griddle or large nonstick frying pan with nonstick
cooking spray. Place over medium-high heat until hot. The
griddle is the right temperature when water dropped on the
surface bounces and dances. If the water evaporates immediately,
the griddle is too hot; if the water sits still, the griddle is not hot
enough. Spoon the batter in scant ⅓-cup (2½-oz/75-g) portions
onto the hot griddle to make 12 pancakes. Flip each pancake
when the surface is covered with tiny bubbles, about 3 minutes.
Cook until the bottom is golden brown, about 2 minutes more.

✳ To serve, divide among 4 individual plates. One serving is
3 pancakes.

Nutritional Analysis per Serving

Calories 298 (Kilojoules 1,252); Total fat 2g; Saturated fat 0g; Protein 10g;
Cholesterol 1mg; Carbohydrates 59g; Sodium 478mg; Dietary fiber 1g;
Calories from fat 6%

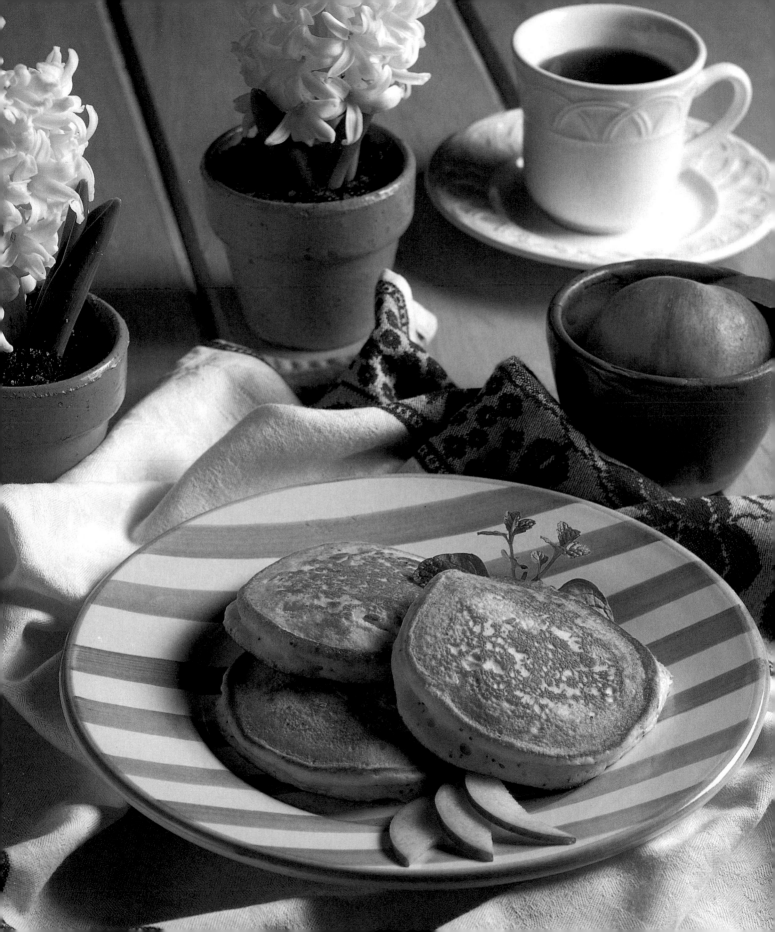

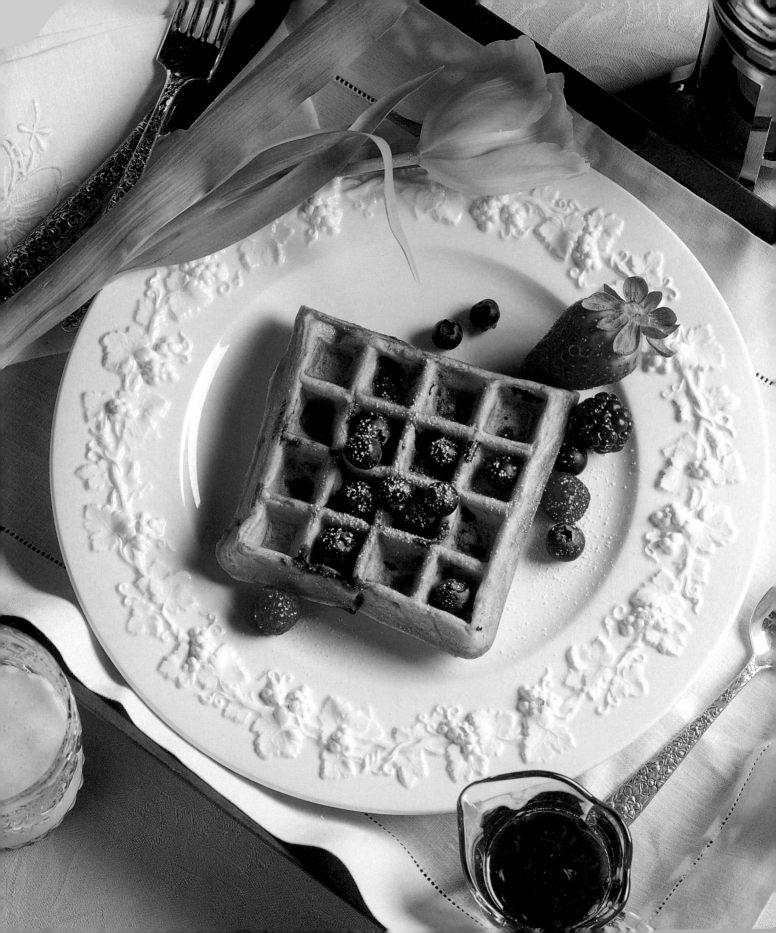

1 cup (5 oz/155 g) unbleached flour

½ cup (2½ oz/75 g) whole wheat (wholemeal) flour

3 tablespoons sugar

1½ teaspoons baking powder

½ teaspoon baking soda (bicarbonate of soda)

¼ teaspoon salt

2 egg whites

1¼ cups (10 fl oz/310 ml) lowfat buttermilk

1 tablespoon margarine, melted

1 teaspoon vanilla extract (essence)

¾ cup (3 oz/90 g) raspberries

¾ cup (3 oz/90 g) blackberries

¾ cup (3 oz/90 g) blueberries

4 strawberries

Cooking Tip

✱ To use the batter for pancakes, omit the fruit and use it all as a topping.

Very Berry Waffles

Preparation: 15 minutes ✱ Cooking: 20 minutes ✱ Serves 4

This topping of seasonal berries adds almost two daily portions of vitamin C- and fiber-rich fruit to each waffle breakfast. In the winter, substitute a different fruit, like sliced bananas or apples, for the berries. If you like, you can spice up the batter with ground cinnamon, nutmeg, cloves or allspice and grated lemon zest.

✱ Coat a waffle iron with nonstick cooking spray and preheat according to the manufacturer's directions.

✱ In a large bowl, combine the flours, sugar, baking powder, baking soda and salt. Make a well in the center. In another large bowl, whisk together the egg whites, buttermilk, margarine and vanilla. Pour the egg white mixture into the well in the flour mixture and stir until just blended. Fold in half each of the raspberries, blackberries and blueberries.

✱ Spoon about 1 cup (8 oz/250 g) of the batter onto the hot waffle iron. Close and cook until golden brown, 4–6 minutes. Repeat with the remaining batter, coating the iron with additional nonstick cooking spray between waffles, as needed, to make 4 waffles. Keep the waffles warm in a 250°F (120°C) oven until all are cooked.

✱ To serve, divide among 4 individual plates. One serving is 1 waffle. Top each with an equal amount of the remaining raspberries, blackberries and blueberries and a strawberry.

Nutritional Analysis per Serving

Calories 336 (Kilojoules 1,411); Total fat 5g; Saturated fat 1g; Protein 11g; Cholesterol 3mg; Carbohydrates 62g; Sodium 619mg; Dietary fiber 6g; Calories from fat 14%

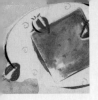

⅔ cup (3 oz/90 g) unbleached flour

⅓ cup (2 oz/60 g) whole wheat (wholemeal) flour

2 tablespoons finely ground cornmeal

2 tablespoons wheat germ

1 teaspoon baking powder

½ teaspoon baking soda (bicarbonate of soda)

3 tablespoons brown sugar

1 teaspoon ground cinnamon

¼ teaspoon salt

1¼ cups (10 fl oz/310 ml) lowfat buttermilk

2 egg whites

1 tablespoon margarine, melted

1 teaspoon vanilla extract (essence)

Cooking Tip

✳ Vigorous mixing of batters with whole wheat flour can tend to make pancakes and baked goods tough. To ensure a tender texture, mix the batter very lightly, just until the ingredients are combined.

Multigrain Pancakes

Preparation: 15 minutes ✳ Cooking: 10 minutes ✳ Serves 4

Each grain contributes different qualities to these pancakes. High-fiber whole wheat flour is milled from the whole kernel. Nutty-tasting wheat germ adds protein, vitamins and minerals. Store these unrefined products in the refrigerator for up to 3 months only. Cornmeal comes in both white and yellow varieties; they are virtually the same for cooking. Look for degerminated and enriched versions, which means the germ has been removed for longer storage but the lost nutrients replaced.

✳ In a large bowl, combine the flours, cornmeal, wheat germ, baking powder, baking soda, brown sugar, cinnamon and salt. Make a well in the center. In another large bowl, whisk together the buttermilk, egg whites, margarine and vanilla. Pour the buttermilk mixture into the well in the flour mixture and stir to mix well.

✳ Coat a griddle or large nonstick frying pan with nonstick cooking spray. Place over medium-high heat until hot. The griddle is the right temperature when water dropped on the surface bounces and dances. If the water evaporates immediately, the griddle is too hot; if the water sits still, the griddle is not hot enough. Spoon the batter in scant ⅓-cup (2½-oz/75-g) portions onto the hot griddle to make 12 pancakes. Flip each pancake when the surface is covered with tiny bubbles, about 4 minutes. Cook until the bottom is golden brown, about 1 minute more.

✳ To serve, divide among 4 individual plates. One serving is 3 pancakes.

Nutritional Analysis per Serving

Calories 267 (Kilojoules 1,122); Total fat 5g; Saturated fat 1g; Protein 10g; Cholesterol 3mg; Carbohydrates 47g; Sodium 561mg; Dietary fiber 3g; Calories from fat 16%

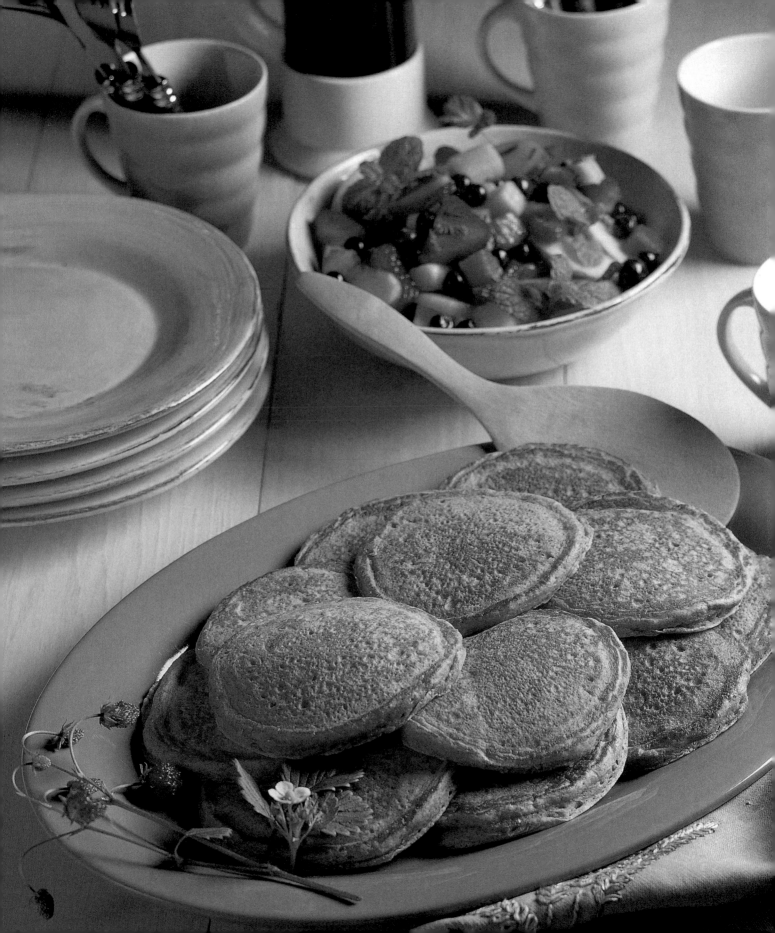

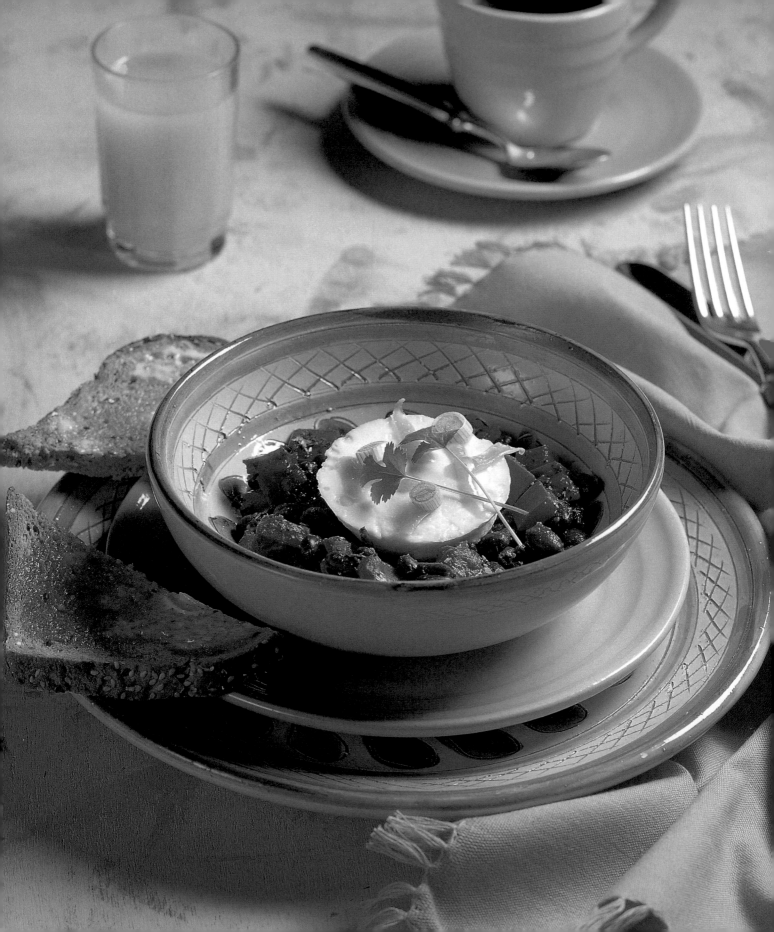

1 cup (7 oz/220 g) dried black beans

4 cups (32 fl oz/1 l) water

1 lb (500 g) whole plum (Roma) tomatoes, chopped

¼ cup (4½ oz/140 g) chopped green chilies

3 teaspoons chili powder

¾ teaspoon ground cumin

½ teaspoon unsweetened Dutch-process cocoa

3 tablespoons chopped fresh cilantro (fresh coriander)

¼ teaspoon ground cayenne pepper

4 eggs

¼ cup (1 oz/30 g) grated reduced fat cheddar cheese

2 tablespoons chopped green (spring) onions, green and white parts

Cooking Tip

✳ If purchasing cooked beans for this recipe, you'll need 2 cups (14 oz/440 g). Be sure to drain and rinse before using. If cooking the beans ahead, cool completely and store in the refrigerator for up to 1 week.

Santa Fe Eggs

Preparation: 10 minutes ✳ *Cooking: 1 hour 25 minutes* ✳ *Serves 4*

Inspired by huevos rancheros, *this dish is reminiscent of the foods I eat when visiting New Mexico. While beans may seem an unlikely breakfast choice, they are a wonderful source of protein and fiber.*

✳ In a large pot over high heat, combine the beans and water and bring to a boil. Reduce the heat to medium and cook for 1 hour, skimming away the gray foam that appears. Drain well.

✳ In a large nonstick frying pan over medium heat, combine the beans, tomatoes, chilies, chili powder, cumin and cocoa. Bring to a boil, reduce the heat to medium-low and simmer until the mixture thickens, about 15 minutes. Stir in the cilantro and cayenne. One at a time, break the eggs into a small bowl and carefully slip on top of the simmering liquid. Cover and poach the eggs until they are just cooked, about 7 minutes. Remove from the heat, sprinkle with the cheese, cover and let stand for 1 minute.

✳ To serve, divide among 4 individual bowls. Top each with an equal amount of the onions.

Nutritional Analysis per Serving

Calories 281 (Kilojoules 1,180); Total fat 8g; Saturated fat 3g; Protein 20g; Cholesterol 218mg; Carbohydrates 36g; Sodium 152mg; Dietary fiber 5g; Calories from fat 24%

1 teaspoon olive oil

1 onion, sliced

1 large green bell pepper (capsicum), seeded, deribbed and sliced into thin strips

½ cup (4 oz/125 g) chopped pimientos (sweet peppers)

1½ cups (9 oz/280 g) corn kernels

½ teaspoon dried oregano

2 eggs

4 egg whites

¼ cup (2 fl oz/60 ml) nonfat milk

¾ teaspoon salt

¼ teaspoon ground black pepper

⅛ teaspoon ground mustard

1 tablespoon grated Romano cheese

Green Pepper-Corn Frittata

*Preparation: 20 minutes * Cooking: 30 minutes * Serves 4*

Bell peppers and corn are excellent sources of vitamin A, and peppers are rich in the antioxidant vitamin C as well. Both vegetables are in season from late spring through early autumn, giving you plenty of opportunity to make this quick meal over and over again.

✳ Preheat an oven to 350°F (180°C). In a large ovenproof frying pan over medium heat, heat the olive oil. Add the onion and green pepper and cook until tender, about 5 minutes. Add the pimientos, corn and oregano and cook for 5 minutes. Transfer the vegetables into a medium bowl.

✳ In a large bowl, combine the eggs, egg whites, milk, salt, pepper and mustard and whisk until blended. Add the egg mixture to the vegetable mixture.

✳ In the same frying pan over low heat, pour in the egg-vegetable mixture. Cook, stirring frequently, until the eggs are firm on the bottom and almost set on the top, 8–10 minutes. Sprinkle the cheese on top and bake in the oven until the eggs are set, 5–8 minutes.

✳ To serve, cut into 4 wedges and divide among individual plates.

Nutritional Analysis per Serving

Calories 160 (Kilojoules 670); Total fat 5g; Saturated fat 1g; Protein 11g; Cholesterol 108mg; Carbohydrates 20g; Sodium 537mg; Dietary fiber 3g; Calories from fat 26%

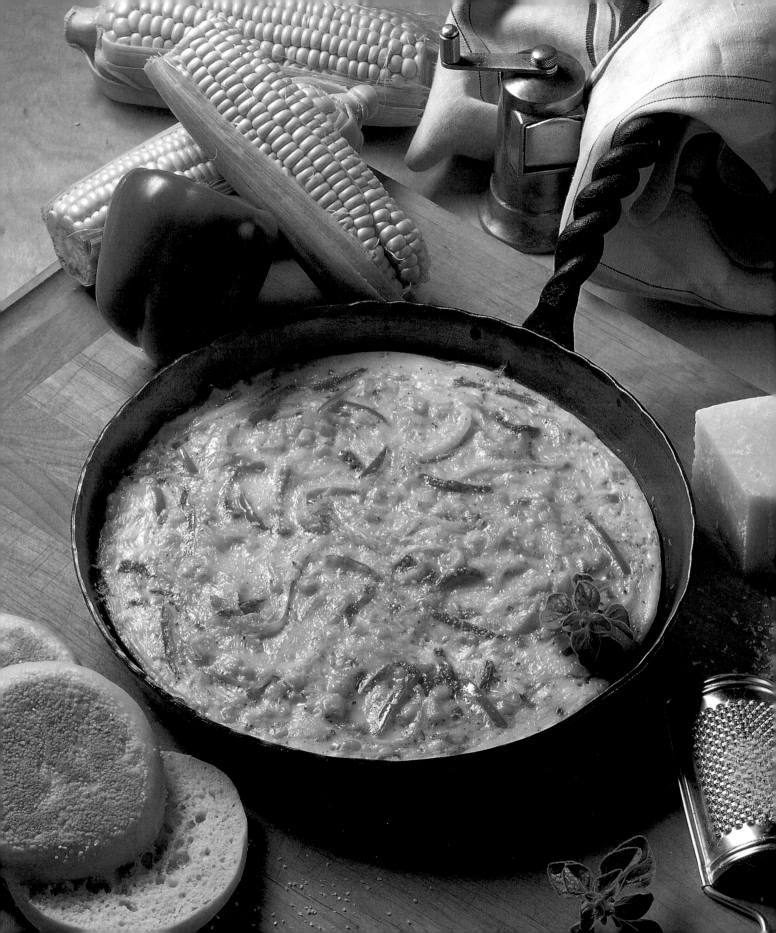

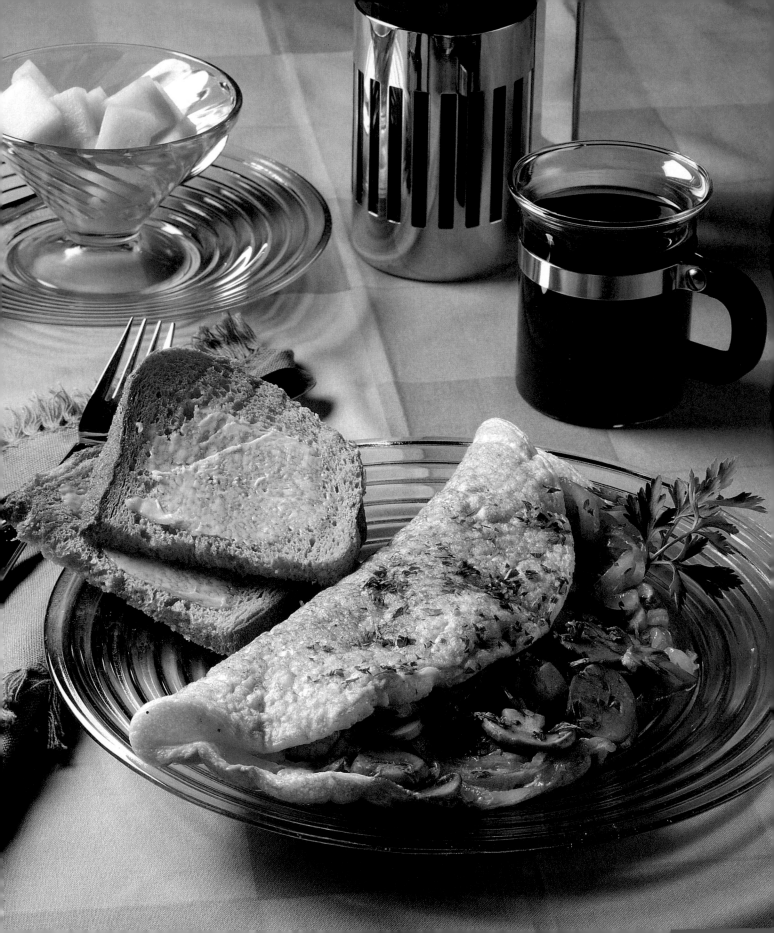

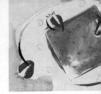

1 teaspoon margarine

1 small onion, thinly sliced

2 teaspoons sugar

1 cup (3 oz/90 g) sliced mushrooms

1 tablespoon balsamic vinegar

3 egg whites

1 tablespoon nonfat milk

¼ teaspoon salt

⅛ teaspoon ground black pepper

1 tablespoon chopped fresh parsley

Nutrition Tip

✳ All the fat and cholesterol in eggs reside in their yolks, while the egg whites are rich in protein and albumin. For healthier cooking of any recipe with eggs, substitute 2 egg whites for each whole egg.

Onion-Mushroom Omelette

*Preparation: 15 minutes * Cooking: 15 minutes * Serves 1*

Healthy diets don't have to be skimpy, as this hearty omelette shows. Designed as a breakfast dish, this works equally well as a light dinner. Containing just 197 calories per serving and requiring only 15 minutes' preparation time, it's a better choice than most "fast food" options.

✳ In a large nonstick frying pan over medium heat, heat the margarine. Add the onion and sugar and cook until the onion is tender and golden brown, about 4 minutes. Add the mushrooms and vinegar and cook until the mushrooms are tender, about 3 minutes. Transfer the onion mixture to a small bowl.

✳ In a large bowl, combine the egg whites, milk, salt and pepper. Using an electric mixer or by hand, beat until stiff peaks form.

✳ Wipe out the frying pan and coat with nonstick cooking spray. Place over medium heat; add the egg-white mixture and gently flatten it using the back of a spoon. Spread the onion mixture over half of the eggs. Cover, reduce the heat to medium-low and cook until the eggs are cooked through and the center of the omelette is set, 4–5 minutes. Using a spatula, carefully loosen the underside of the omelette, fold in half, cover and cook for 1 minute more.

✳ To serve, slide the omelette onto a plate and garnish with the parsley. If preparing several omelettes, keep the first ones warm, covered with foil, in a 250°F (120°C) oven until all are cooked.

Nutritional Analysis per Serving

Calories 197 (Kilojoules 827); Total fat 5g; Saturated fat 1g; Protein 14g; Cholesterol 0mg; Carbohydrates 25g; Sodium 766mg; Dietary fiber 3g; Calories from fat 24%

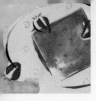

⅛ lb (60 g) Canadian bacon,
    cut into 4 slices

4 eggs

4 English muffins, halved and toasted

½ teaspoon ground paprika

Lowfat Hollandaise

⅔ cup (5 fl oz/160 ml) nonfat
    evaporated milk

1 egg yolk

¼ teaspoon salt

2 teaspoons margarine

1 tablespoon unbleached flour

1 tablespoon lemon juice

Nutrition Tip

✳ To lower the percentage of calories from
fat for your meal as a whole, pair Eggs
Benedict with Rosemary Roasted Potatoes
(recipe on page 202) as outlined in the
Suggested Menu on page 35.

Eggs Benedict with Lowfat Hollandaise

Preparation: 25 minutes ✳ *Cooking: 15 minutes* ✳ *Serves 4*

*I'm very fond of eggs Benedict and asked Robin Vitetta to develop a
healthy version. This is the most nutritious recipe we could come up with
that still tastes the way the dish ought to taste. It is still higher in fat than
our healthy goals and for that reason should be eaten as a special-occasion
treat. Consider it for brunch, after an all-fruit breakfast, and plan an
especially lowfat dinner that evening.*

✳ Coat a large nonstick frying pan with nonstick cooking spray
and place over medium heat. Add the Canadian bacon and cook
until brown on both sides, 3 minutes. Drain on paper towels.

✳ In a medium saucepan over high heat, bring 4 inches (10 cm)
of water to a boil. Reduce the heat to medium–low. One at a
time, break the eggs into a small bowl and carefully slip into the
simmering water. Poach until the whites are cooked through,
3–5 minutes.

✳ To serve, stack 2 English muffin halves on 4 individual plates.
Top each stack with 1 slice of Canadian bacon. Using a slotted
spoon, place an egg on top of the bacon. Top each with an equal
amount of the Lowfat Hollandaise and paprika.

Lowfat Hollandaise

✳ In a small bowl, whisk together the milk, egg yolk and salt.
In a nonstick frying pan over medium heat, heat the margarine.
Gradually whisk in the flour, reduce the heat to low and cook,
stirring constantly, until smooth and bubbly, about 3 minutes.

✳ Increase the heat to medium. Gradually add the milk mixture,
stirring constantly, and bring to a boil. Reduce the heat to low and
simmer, stirring constantly, until thick and bubbly, about 1 minute.
Remove from the heat and stir in the lemon juice.

Nutritional Analysis per Serving

Calories 306 (Kilojoules 1,287); Total fat 11g; Saturated fat 3g; Protein 18g;
Cholesterol 274mg; Carbohydrates 34g; Sodium 736mg; Dietary fiber 1g;
Calories from fat 32%

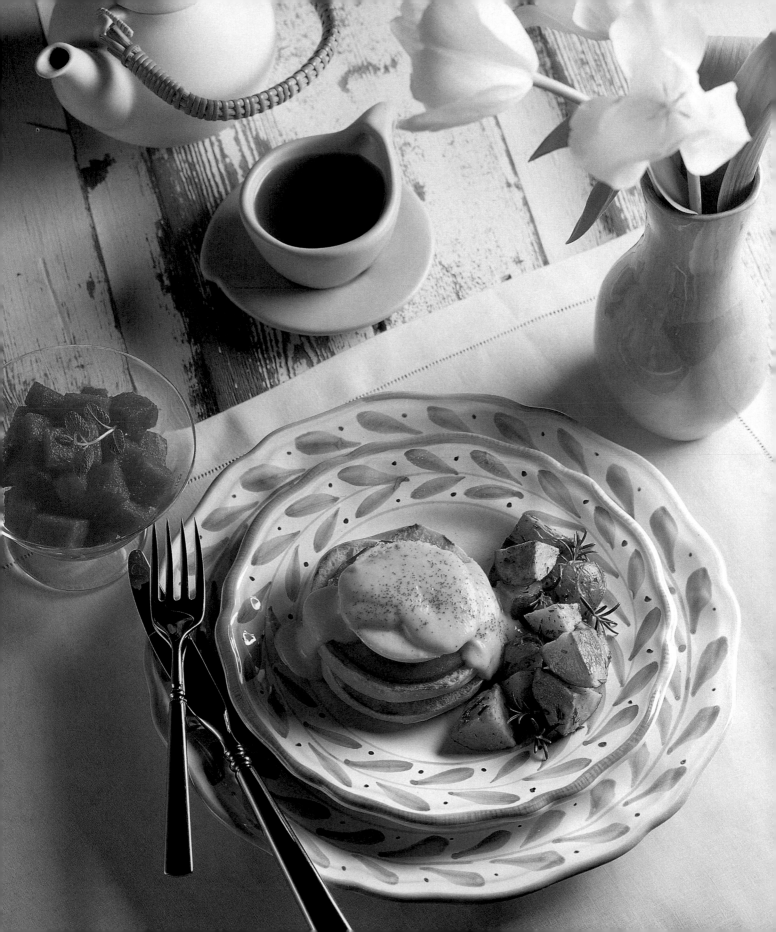

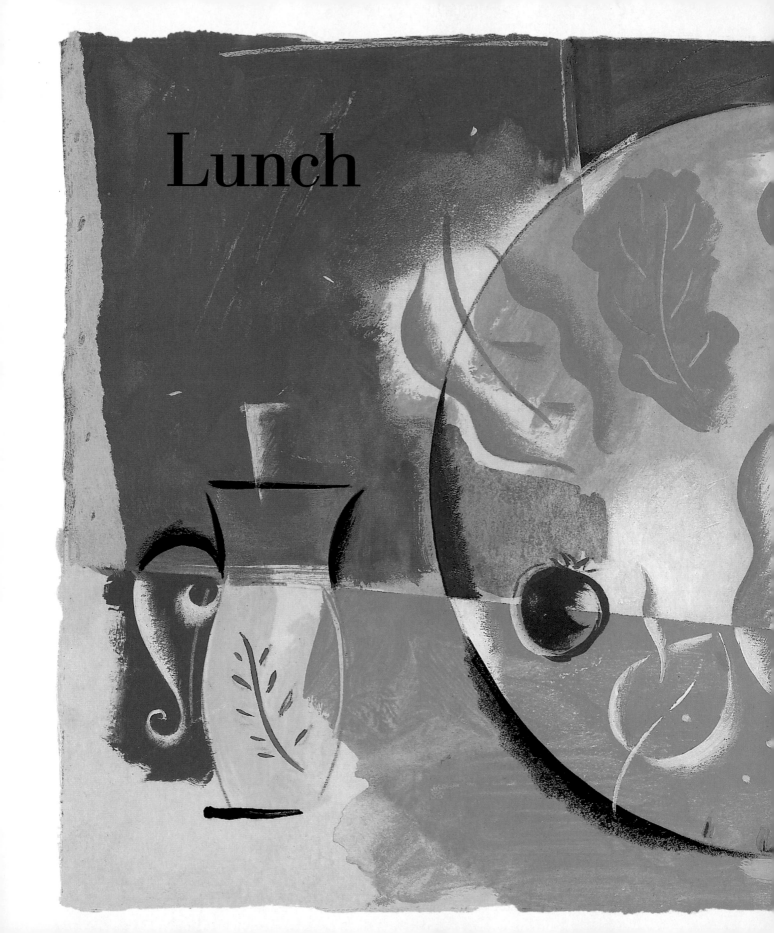

Lunch

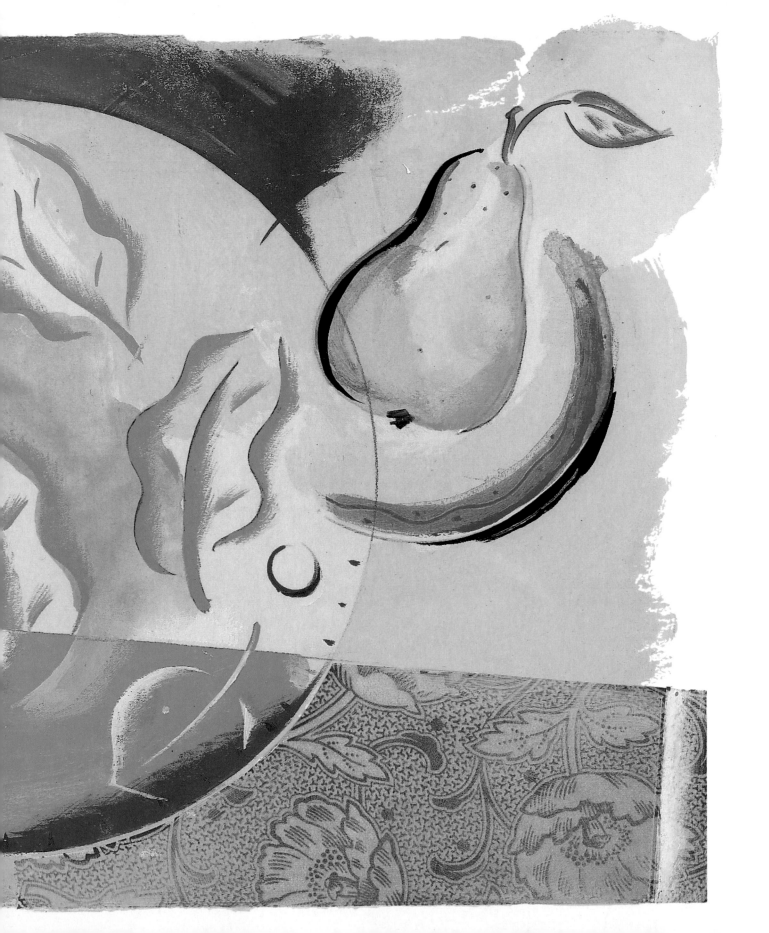

Suggested Lunch Menus

With the busy lives so many of us lead today, lunch all too often gets short shrift as a quickly eaten fast-food meal. That's a shame, because midday is the time for most efficiently supplying our bodies with the proteins we need, accompanied by complex carbohydrates for sustained energy. The menus shown here and the recipes on the pages that follow, however, demonstrate how simple it can be to prepare your own healthy lunch that is easy to eat, completely satisfying and full of foods that are high in flavor and low in fat. Many of them also pack easily, allowing you to enjoy a healthy meal even in the midst of the most hectic day.

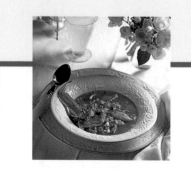

Louisiana Crab Gumbo
page 84

Caponata
page 189

1 apple

8 fl oz (250 ml) lemonade

Nutritional Analysis per Serving: Calories 596 (Kilojoules 2,503); Total fat 9g; Saturated fat 1g; Protein 30g; Cholesterol 85mg; Carbohydrates 106g; Sodium 990mg; Dietary fiber 16g; Calories from fat 13%

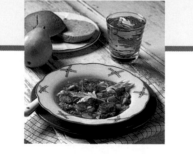

Turkey-Vegetable Gumbo
page 87

1 whole wheat roll

1 pear

herbal iced tea

Nutritional Analysis per Serving: Calories 482 (Kilojoules 2,024); Total fat 7g; Saturated fat 2g; Protein 18g; Cholesterol 15mg; Carbohydrates 91g; Sodium 1,239mg; Dietary fiber 18g; Calories from fat 13%

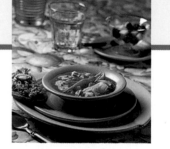

Hearty Vegetable Stew
page 88

Mushroom-Topped Crostini
page 190

¼ cup (1 oz/30 g) blackberries and ¼ cantaloupe

mineral water

Nutritional Analysis per Serving: Calories 500 (Kilojoules 2,099); Total fat 8g; Saturated fat 1g; Protein 17g; Cholesterol 0mg; Carbohydrates 95g; Sodium 1,122mg; Dietary fiber 14g; Calories from fat 15%

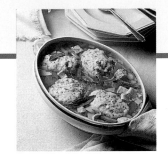

Chicken Soup
with Parsley Dumplings
page 91

1 carrot and 1 celery stalk
with Chive-Chutney Dip
page 186

6 fl oz (185 ml) cranberry juice
with 2 fl oz (60 ml) seltzer water

Nutritional Analysis per Serving: Calories 592
(Kilojoules 2,486); Total fat 5g; Saturated fat 1g;
Protein 39g; Cholesterol 82mg; Carbohydrates 95g;
Sodium 1,444mg; Dietary fiber 7g; Calories from fat 7%

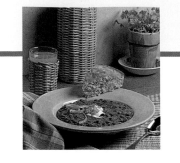

Black Bean Soup
page 92

Chili-Cheese Corn Bread
page 193

Iced Fruit Cider
page 180

Nutritional Analysis per Serving: Calories 843
(Kilojoules 3,542); Total fat 8g; Saturated fat 1g;
Protein 34g; Cholesterol 1mg; Carbohydrates 163g;
Sodium 698mg; Dietary fiber 19g; Calories from fat 8%

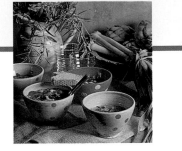

Pasta and Watercress Soup
page 95

2 slices whole wheat bread
with 2 teaspoons cream cheese

1 peach

8 fl oz (250 ml) grape juice

Nutritional Analysis per Serving: Calories 689
(Kilojoules 2,892); Total fat 10g; Saturated fat 3g;
Protein 19g; Cholesterol 10mg; Carbohydrates 138g;
Sodium 408mg; Dietary fiber 11g; Calories from fat 12%

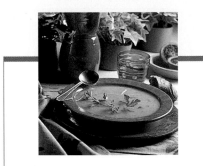

Potato Soup
page 96

2 slices dark rye bread

1 orange

mineral water

Nutritional Analysis per Serving: Calories 442
(Kilojoules 1,856); Total fat 4g; Saturated fat 1g;
Protein 15mg; Cholesterol 1mg; Carbohydrates 85g;
Sodium 1,264g; Dietary fiber 12g; Calories from fat 9%

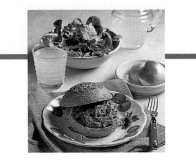

Shredded Chicken Sandwich
page 99

1 cup (2 oz/60 g) mixed greens
with Mustard Vinaigrette
page 184

1 nectarine

8 fl oz (250 ml) lemonade

Nutritional Analysis per Serving: Calories 545
(Kilojoules 2,287); Total fat 6g; Saturated fat 1g;
Protein 35g; Cholesterol 1mg; Carbohydrates 91g;
Sodium 1,035g; Dietary fiber 9g; Calories from fat 10%

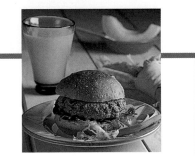

Spicy Chicken Burgers
with Creamy Horseradish
page 100

1 tomato and ½ cucumber sliced
with Dill Dressing
page 183

¼ honeydew melon

6 fl oz (185 ml) orange juice
with 2 fl oz (60 ml) seltzer water

Nutritional Analysis per Serving: Calories 535
(Kilojoules 2,246); Total fat 5g; Saturated fat 1g;
Protein 40g; Cholesterol 67mg; Carbohydrates 88g;
Sodium 611mg; Dietary fiber 9g; Calories from fat 8%

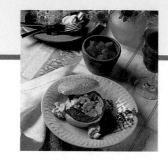

*Turkey Burgers
with Mushroom Sauce*
page 103

*1 cup (2 oz/60 g) mixed greens
with Basil Dressing*
page 183

*1 cup (6 oz/185 g)
watermelon chunks*

Tangy Tomato Drink
page 180

Nutritional Analysis per Serving: Calories 460
(Kilojoules 1,932); Total fat 6g; Saturated fat 1g;
Protein 43g; Cholesterol 71mg; Carbohydrates 61g;
Sodium 671mg; Dietary fiber 4g; Calories from fat 11%

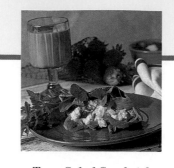

Tuna Salad Sandwich
page 104

*½ cup (4 oz/125 g) nonfat
plain yogurt*

½ cup (2 oz/60 g) strawberries

Iced Skinny Café Mocha
page 179

Nutritional Analysis per Serving: Calories 406
(Kilojoules 1,704); Total fat 5g; Saturated fat 2g;
Protein 37g; Cholesterol 38mg; Carbohydrates 54g;
Sodium 799mg; Dietary fiber 6g; Calories from fat 10%

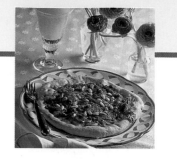

Tomato-Basil Pizza
page 107

1 cup (6 oz/185 g) green grapes

8 fl oz (250 ml) grapefruit juice

Nutritional Analysis per Serving: Calories 826
(Kilojoules 3,468); Total fat 15g; Saturated fat 2g;
Protein 26g; Cholesterol 4mg; Carbohydrates 156g;
Sodium 840mg; Dietary fiber 18g; Calories from fat 16%

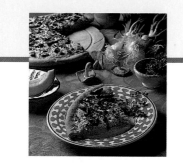

Mushroom-Cheese Pizza
page 108

¼ cantaloupe

8 fl oz (250 ml) apple juice

Nutritional Analysis per Serving: Calories 705
(Kilojoules 2,963); Total fat 14g; Saturated fat 2g;
Protein 20g; Cholesterol 7mg; Carbohydrates 130g;
Sodium 803mg; Dietary fiber 12g; Calories from fat 17%

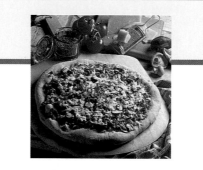

Ted's Favorite Pizza
page 111

Tangy Tomato Drink
page 180

Nutritional Analysis per Serving: Calories 750
(Kilojoules 3,148); Total fat 17g; Saturated fat 5g;
Protein 44g; Cholesterol 51mg; Carbohydrates 114g;
Sodium 1,516mg; Dietary fiber 14g; Calories from fat 19%

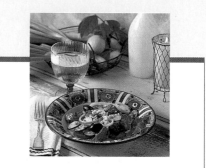

Greek Salad
page 112

Baked French Fries
page 202

1 apple

mineral water

Nutritional Analysis per Serving: Calories 469
(Kilojoules 1,971); Total fat 16g; Saturated fat 5g;
Protein 26g; Cholesterol 59mg; Carbohydrates 60g;
Sodium 813mg; Dietary fiber 8g; Calories from fat 29%

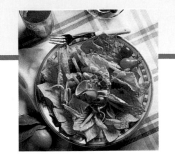

*Taco Salad
with Avocado Dressing*
page 115

1 carrot

4 Kalamata olives

*4 fl oz (125 ml) orange juice
with 4 fl oz (125 ml) seltzer water*

Nutritional Analysis per Serving: Calories 396
(Kilojoules 1,663); Total fat 15g; Saturated fat 2g;
Protein 11g; Cholesterol 1mg; Carbohydrates 57g;
Sodium 606mg; Dietary fiber 8g; Calories from fat 34%

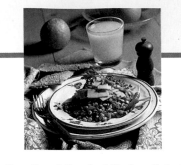

Lentil and Smoked Turkey Salad
page 116

2 flatbread crackers

1 orange

8 fl oz (250 ml) grapefruit juice

Nutritional Analysis per Serving: Calories 621
(Kilojoules 2,610); Total fat 8g; Saturated fat 1g;
Protein 34g; Cholesterol 18mg; Carbohydrates 107g;
Sodium 113mg; Dietary fiber 17g; Calories from fat 12%

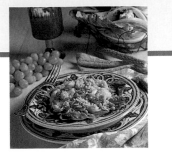

*Curried Chicken, Rice
and Spinach Salad*
page 119

2 sesame bread sticks

½ cup (3 oz/90 g) green grapes

Tangy Tomato Drink
page 180

Nutritional Analysis per Serving: Calories 551
(Kilojoules 2,314); Total fat 8g; Saturated fat 1g;
Protein 44g; Cholesterol 66mg; Carbohydrates 82g;
Sodium 1,038mg; Dietary fiber 9g; Calories from fat 13%

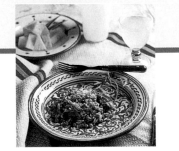

*Orzo, Sun-Dried Tomato
and Pea Salad*
page 120

*5 melba toast crackers
with Creamy Spinach Spread*
page 186

*1 cup (6 oz/185 g)
pineapple chunks*

8 fl oz (250 ml) lemonade

Nutritional Analysis per Serving: Calories 663
(Kilojoules 2,787); Total fat 7g; Saturated fat 1g;
Protein 22g; Cholesterol 4mg; Carbohydrates 132g;
Sodium 536mg; Dietary fiber 10g; Calories from fat 9%

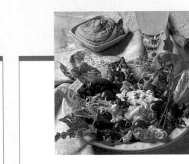

Tabbouleh
page 123

Chili-Cheese Corn Bread
page 193

1 apple

Iced Fruit Cider
page 180

Nutritional Analysis per Serving: Calories 739
(Kilojoules 3,106); Total fat 17g; Saturated fat 2g;
Protein 16g; Cholesterol 1mg; Carbohydrates 139g;
Sodium 813mg; Dietary fiber 17g; Calories from fat 20%

Greens and Peppers Salad
page 124

Hummus with Pita Bread
page 190

mineral water

Nutritional Analysis per Serving: Calories 282
(Kilojoules 1,184); Total fat 4g; Saturated fat 2g;
Protein 12g; Cholesterol 5mg; Carbohydrates 50g;
Sodium 416mg; Dietary fiber 4g; Calories from fat 13%

2 teaspoons vegetable oil

1 large onion, chopped

3 garlic cloves, peeled and minced

2 celery stalks, sliced crosswise

1 green bell pepper (capsicum),
seeded, deribbed and chopped

1½ cups (12 fl oz/375 ml) Chicken
Stock (recipe on page 206) or
reduced sodium chicken broth

3 large tomatoes, peeled, seeded
and diced

1 cup (8 fl oz/250 ml) bottled
clam juice

1 tablespoon chopped fresh oregano

1 bay leaf

¼ teaspoon hot pepper sauce

¼ teaspoon ground black pepper

2 cups (12 oz/375 g) sliced okra

2 cups (12 oz/375 g) cooked,
shredded crabmeat, picked
over to remove shells

1 cup (6 oz/185 g) corn kernels

Louisiana Crab Gumbo

*Preparation: 20 minutes * Cooking: 25 minutes * Serves 4*

Okra, native to Africa, is used extensively in Creole cooking. In fact, the term gumbo *is derived from an African word for the plant. The slender, ribbed or smooth, fuzzy, green pods are 1 to 3 inches (2.5 to 7.5 cm) long and have a mild flavor resembling that of green beans. Okra can be blanched and served cold in salads, sautéed and served as a side dish or used as a thickener in soups and stews.*

✳ In a large saucepan over medium heat, heat the oil. Add the onion, garlic, celery and green pepper and sauté until tender, about 5 minutes.

✳ Add the stock or broth, tomatoes, clam juice, oregano, bay leaf, hot sauce and pepper and bring to a boil. Add the okra, crabmeat and corn, reduce the heat to low and simmer, stirring frequently, until the gumbo thickens, about 10 minutes. Remove and discard the bay leaf.

✳ To serve, divide among 4 individual bowls.

Nutritional Analysis per Serving

Calories 243 (Kilojoules 1,021); Total fat 5g; Saturated fat 1g; Protein 23g; Cholesterol 85mg; Carbohydrates 28g; Sodium 628mg; Dietary fiber 7g; Calories from fat 18%

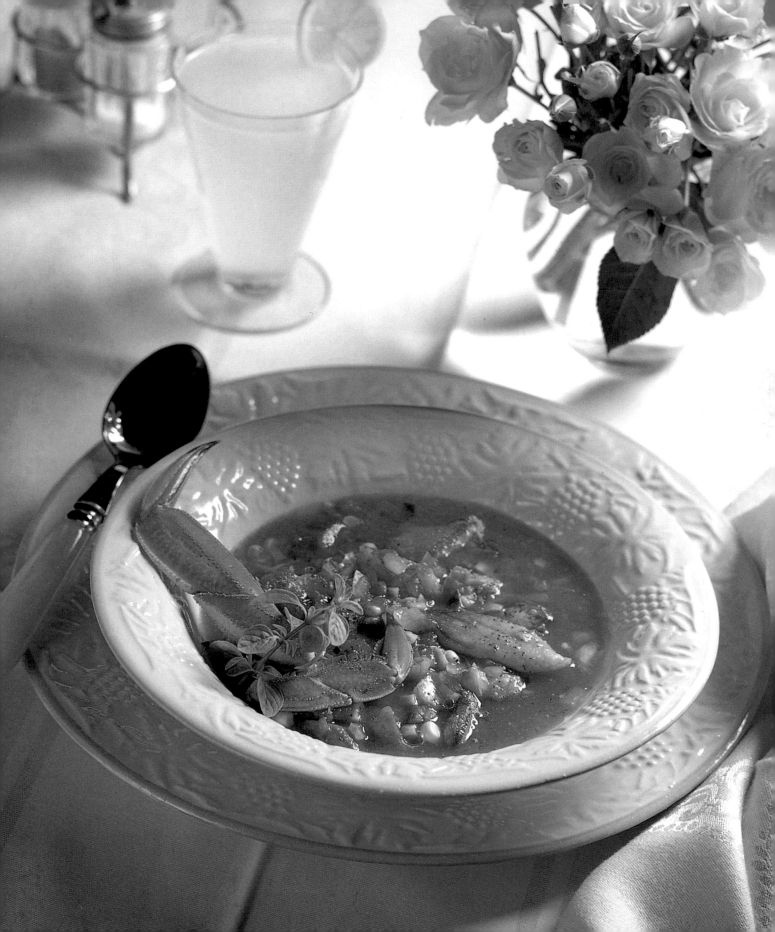

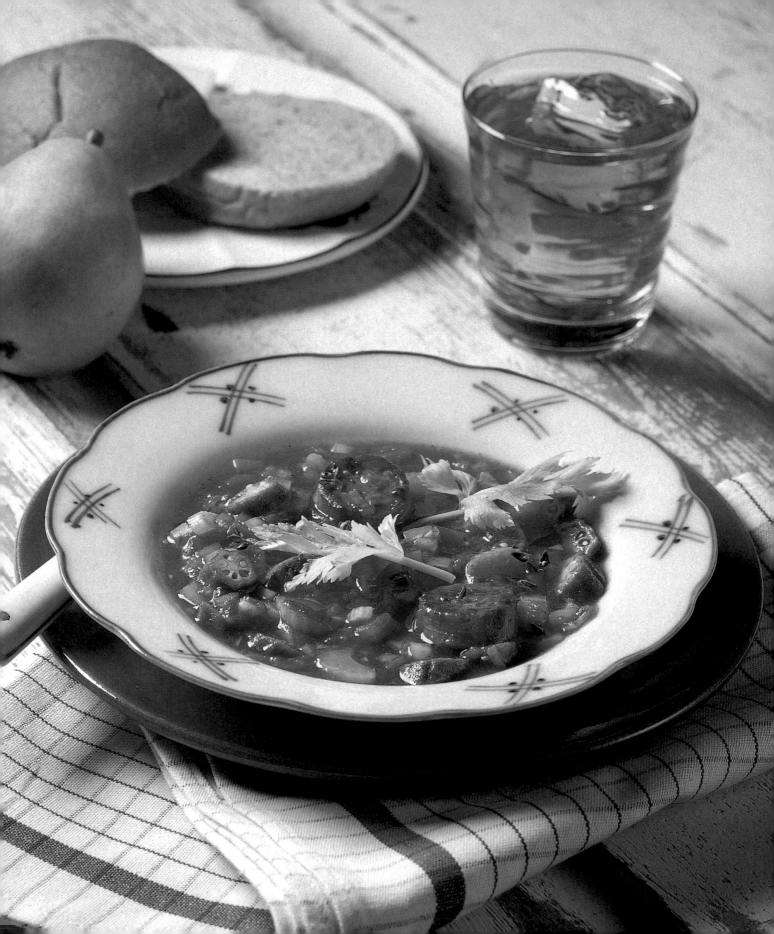

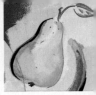

Turkey-Vegetable Gumbo

4 oz (125 g) turkey sausages, cut
   into 1-inch (2.5-cm) slices

1 onion, chopped

2 garlic cloves, peeled and minced

2 celery stalks, sliced crosswise

1 red bell pepper (capsicum), seeded,
   deribbed and chopped

2 teaspoons chili powder

1 tablespoon chopped fresh thyme

1 tablespoon chopped fresh oregano

1 bay leaf

½ teaspoon salt

¼ teaspoon hot pepper sauce

2 cups (12 oz/375 g) sliced okra

3 large tomatoes, peeled, seeded
   and diced

½ cup (3 oz/90 g) uncooked
   pearl barley

3 cups (24 fl oz/750 ml) Chicken
   Stock (recipe on page 206) or
   reduced sodium chicken broth

Preparation: 30 minutes ✱ Cooking: 45 minutes ✱ Serves 4

This thick soup is a good example of using animal protein—here, turkey sausage—as a flavoring element in a dish rather than as the center of the meal. Sautéing the vegetables with the meat and then simmering them in the broth provides the desired spicy sausage taste, but each serving contains only 1 oz (30 g) of meat, which is well within healthy eating guidelines.

✱ Coat a large nonstick saucepan with nonstick cooking spray and place over medium heat. Add the sausage and sauté until browned all over and no longer pink in the center, about 5 minutes. Add the onion, garlic, celery and bell pepper. Sauté until the vegetables are tender, about 5 minutes.

✱ Add the chili powder, thyme, oregano, bay leaf, salt, hot pepper sauce, okra, tomatoes, barley and stock or broth and bring to a boil. Reduce the heat to low and simmer, stirring frequently, until the gumbo thickens and the barley is tender, about 30 minutes. Remove and discard the bay leaf.

✱ To serve, divide among 4 individual bowls.

Storage Tip

✱ Store this soup in an airtight container in the refrigerator for up to 3 days or in the freezer for up to 3 months.

Nutritional Analysis per Serving

Calories 241 (Kilojoules 1,012); Total fat 4g; Saturated fat 1g; Protein 12g; Cholesterol 15mg; Carbohydrates 39g; Sodium 938mg; Dietary fiber 10g; Calories from fat 16%

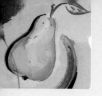

2 teaspoons olive oil

1 onion, chopped

½ head green cabbage
(about 8 oz/250 g), cut into
2-inch (5-cm) pieces

2 carrots, cut into 1-inch (2.5-cm)
pieces

2 celery stalks, cut into 1-inch
(2.5-cm) pieces

1 zucchini (courgette), cut into 1-inch
(2.5-cm) pieces

4 small red potatoes (about 1 lb/500 g),
peels intact, cut into 1-inch
(2.5-cm) pieces

8 oz (250 g) fresh mushrooms, sliced

6 tomatoes, peeled, seeded and diced

1¾ cups (14 fl oz/440 ml) Chicken
Stock (recipe on page 206) or
reduced sodium chicken broth

¼ cup (½ oz/15 g) chopped fresh
basil

1 tablespoon chopped fresh thyme

½ teaspoon salt

¼ teaspoon ground black pepper

Hearty Vegetable Stew

Preparation: 20 minutes ✳ Cooking: 45 minutes ✳ Serves 4

This combination of winter vegetables is a rich source of antioxidants, getting vitamin C from cabbage and tomatoes and beta-carotene from the carrots. It makes a perfect choice for a lunch to go. If you have facilities for reheating, just pack portions in an airtight container. If not, invest in a wide-mouth vacuum bottle, and you can look forward to your healthy lunch all morning long. Use the time you save by not going out for lunch to take a brisk walk.

✳ In a large stockpot over medium heat, heat the oil. Add the onion and cabbage and sauté until tender, about 5 minutes. Add the carrots, celery, zucchini, potatoes and mushrooms and sauté for 5 minutes.

✳ Add the tomatoes, stock or broth, basil, thyme, salt and pepper. Bring to a boil, reduce the heat to low and simmer until the potatoes are tender, about 30 minutes.

✳ To serve, divide among 4 individual bowls.

Nutritional Analysis per Serving

Calories 232 (Kilojoules 973); Total fat 4g; Saturated fat 0g; Protein 8g; Cholesterol 0mg; Carbohydrates 45g; Sodium 589mg; Dietary fiber 9g; Calories from fat 13%

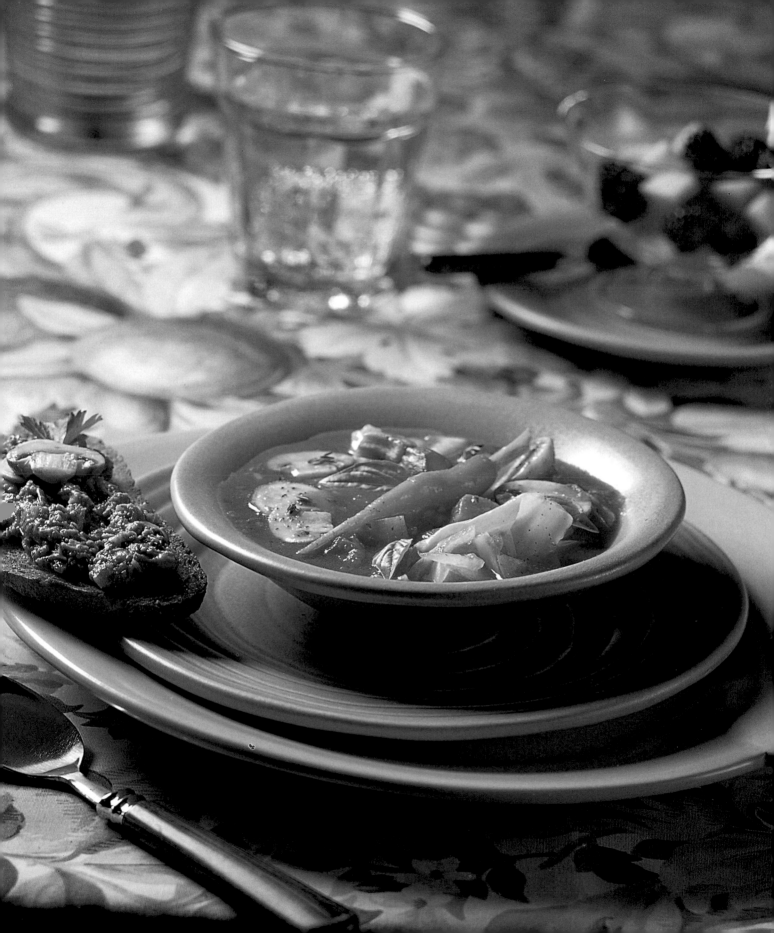

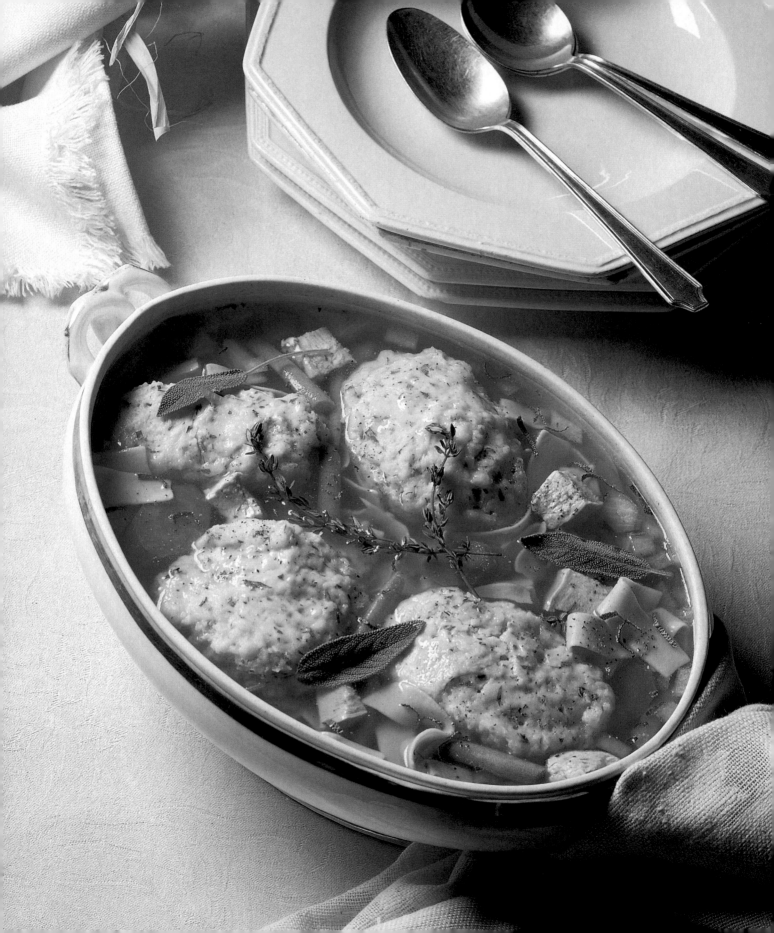

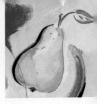

12 oz (375 g) skinless, boneless
   chicken breast
3½ cups (28 fl oz/875 ml) Chicken
   Stock (recipe on page 206) or
   reduced sodium chicken broth
1½ cups (12 fl oz/375 ml) water
2 bay leaves
1 tablespoon chopped fresh thyme
1 teaspoon chopped fresh sage
¼ teaspoon ground black pepper
½ teaspoon salt
1 onion, chopped
2 carrots, cut into ½-inch (12-mm)
   thick slices
8 oz (250 g) green beans, trimmed
4 oz (125 g) dried egg noodles
½ cup (2½ oz/75 g) unbleached flour
2 tablespoons chopped fresh flat-leaf
   (Italian) parsley
¾ teaspoon baking powder
⅛ teaspoon baking soda
   (bicarbonate of soda)
⅛ teaspoon ground white pepper
1½ teaspoons margarine
¼ cup (2 fl oz/60 ml) lowfat
   buttermilk
1 egg white

Cooking Tip

✳ Make the dumplings just before placing
them on the hot soup to prevent the
baking powder from rising too soon.

Chicken Soup with Parsley Dumplings

Preparation: 30 minutes ✳ *Cooking: 20 minutes* ✳ *Serves 4*

*Carrots, green beans and fresh herbs give this chicken noodle soup color
and flavor; the parsley dumplings make it a meal in a bowl. If you have it
available, substitute 2 cups (12 oz/375 g) of cooked chicken for the breast.*

✳ To make the soup, in a medium saucepan over medium-high
heat, poach the chicken breast in 1 inch (2.5 cm) of water until
it is no longer pink in the center, about 10 minutes. Transfer to a
work surface and cut into bite-sized pieces.

✳ In a large saucepan over medium heat, combine the stock or
broth, water, bay leaves, thyme, sage, black pepper and half the
salt and bring to a boil. Add the onion, carrots, green beans,
noodles and cooked chicken. Return to a boil, reduce the heat
to low and simmer until the carrots are tender, about 3 minutes.

✳ To make the dumplings, in a large bowl, combine the flour,
parsley, baking powder, baking soda, remaining salt and white
pepper. Add the margarine and, using a fork, stir until the mixture
resembles coarse meal. In a small bowl, combine the buttermilk
and egg white and whisk until blended. Add to the flour mixture
and stir until just blended.

✳ Divide the dough into 4 pieces and gently place on top of
the soup. Simmer, covered, until the dumplings are puffed up,
10–12 minutes. Remove and discard the bay leaves.

✳ To serve, place one dumpling in each of 4 bowls and top each
with an equal amount of the soup.

Nutritional Analysis per Serving

Calories 371 (Kilojoules 1,557); Total fat 4g; Saturated fat 1g; Protein 31g;
Cholesterol 77mg; Carbohydrates 49g; Sodium 1,020mg; Dietary fiber 4g;
Calories from fat 11%

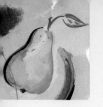

2 cups (14 oz/440 g) dried black beans

8 cups (64 fl oz/2 l) water

8 cups (64 fl oz/2 l) Vegetable
Stock (recipe on page 207) or
vegetable broth

1 large onion, chopped

2 garlic cloves, peeled and minced

2 carrots, sliced in ½-inch (12-mm)
pieces

1½ teaspoons ground cumin

1 teaspoon chili powder

¼ cup (2 fl oz/60 ml) orange juice

¼ cup (⅓ oz/10 g) chopped fresh
cilantro (fresh coriander)

½ cup (4 oz/125 g) nonfat dairy
sour cream

Cooking Tip

✳ You may find it easiest simply to soak the beans overnight in water to cover, drain them and begin making the soup at the second step. If you prefer a smooth texture, purée all the soup in the fourth step.

Black Bean Soup

Preparation: 20 minutes ✳ *Cooking: 2 hours 30 minutes* ✳ *Serves 4*

This filling, flavorful soup is completely vegetarian and very low in fat, but I have to admit a preference for a delicious meat version. I add 4 oz (125 g) chopped chorizo, a cooked pork sausage, along with the onion. The nutritional analysis of that version: calories 583 (kilojoules 2,450), total fat 12g, saturated fat 3g, protein 32g, cholesterol 24mg, carbohydrates 89g, sodium 558mg, dietary fiber 15g, and calories from fat 18%.

✳ In a large pot over high heat, combine the beans and water and bring to a boil. Reduce the heat to medium and cook for 10 minutes, skimming away the gray foam that appears. Drain well.

✳ In a large stockpot over medium heat, combine the beans and stock or broth and bring to a boil. Reduce the heat to low and simmer for 1½ hours.

✳ Coat a large nonstick frying pan with nonstick cooking spray and place over medium heat. Add the onion and garlic and sauté until the onion is tender, about 5 minutes. Stir the onion mixture into the beans. Add the carrots, cumin, chili powder and orange juice. Simmer for 45 minutes.

✳ Remove 1 cup (8 oz/250 g) of the mixture, place in a food processor with the metal blade or in a blender, purée until smooth and return to the pot. Remove from the heat and stir in half the cilantro.

✳ To serve, divide among 4 individual bowls. Top each with an equal amount of the sour cream and remaining cilantro.

Nutritional Analysis per Serving

Calories 479 (Kilojoules 2,010); Total fat 3g; Saturated fat 0g; Protein 27g; Cholesterol 0mg; Carbohydrates 89g; Sodium 191mg; Dietary fiber 15g; Calories from fat 5%

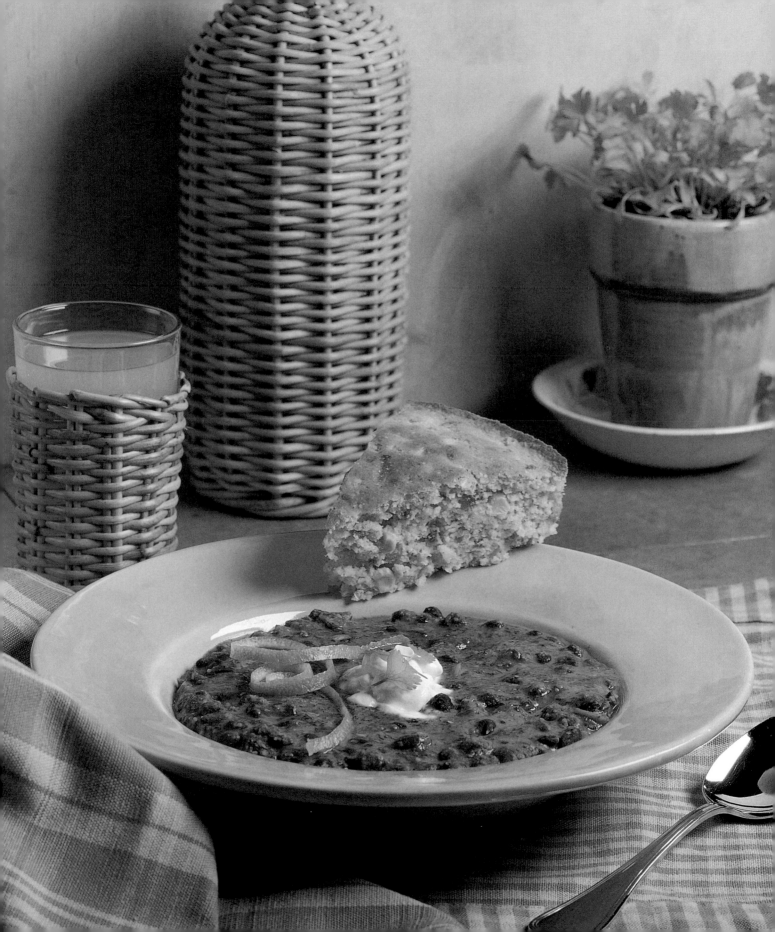

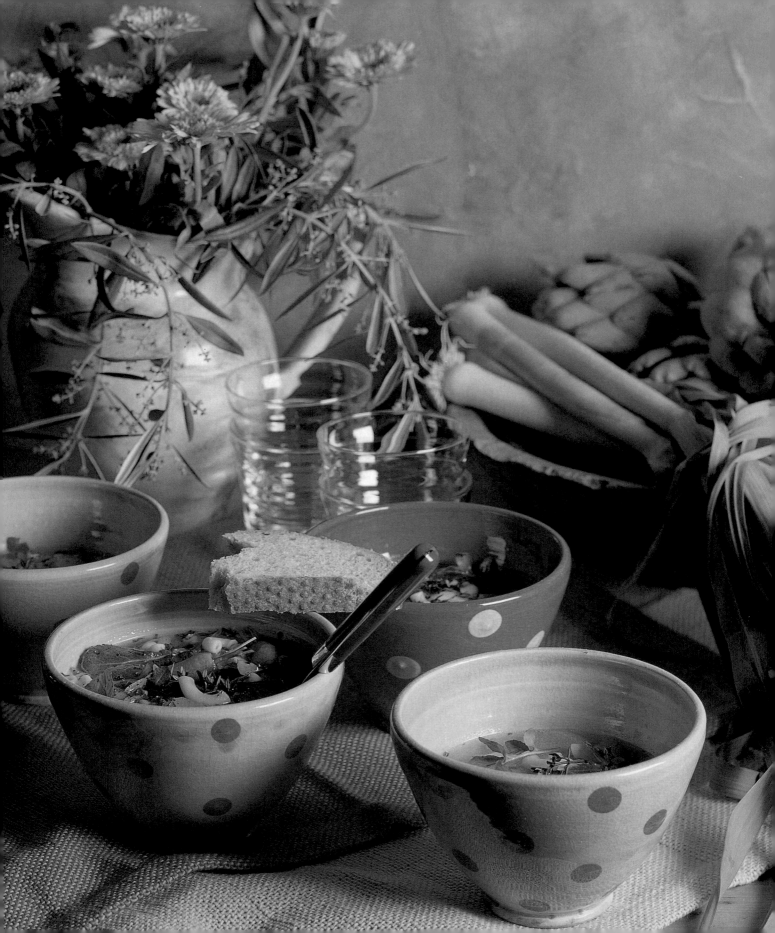

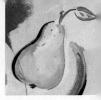

2 teaspoons olive oil

2 leeks, green and white parts,
finely chopped

2 carrots, peeled and chopped

6 cups (48 fl oz/1.5 l) Vegetable
Stock (recipe on page 207) or
vegetable broth

¼ cup (⅓ oz/10 g) chopped
fresh thyme

2 tablespoons chopped fresh oregano

8 oz (250 g) dried elbow pasta

8 oz (250 g) watercress, stemmed

¼ teaspoon ground black pepper

Cooking Tip

✳ To chop fresh herbs, rinse them under
cold running water and dry thoroughly
by shaking or gently patting with kitchen
towels. If leaves are attached to woody
stems, pull them off. Gather the leaves
into a compact bunch and, with a sharp
knife, carefully cut crosswise to chop
coarsely. Chop further if a finer consistency
is required.

Pasta and Watercress Soup

Preparation: 20 minutes ✳ Cooking: 45 minutes ✳ Serves 4

*Peppery-tasting watercress, a member of the mustard family that packs
a good amount of vitamin C, has small, dark green leaves on a stem
slightly thicker than that of parsley. It's usually available commercially
all year. If you're growing it in your herb garden, water it generously
and expect peak supplies in late spring.*

✳ In a large saucepan over medium heat, heat the oil. Add the
leeks and carrots and sauté, stirring frequently, until tender, about
10 minutes.

✳ Add the stock or broth, thyme and oregano, increase the heat
to medium-high and bring to a boil.

✳ Reduce the heat to low, cover and simmer for 20 minutes.

✳ Uncover, increase the heat to medium-high and bring to a
boil. Add the pasta and watercress and cook according to the
package directions or until the pasta is al dente, about 10 minutes.
Add the pepper.

✳ To serve, divide among 4 individual bowls.

Nutritional Analysis per Serving

Calories 332 (Kilojoules 1,396); Total fat 4g; Saturated fat 1g; Protein 11g;
Cholesterol 0mg; Carbohydrates 65g; Sodium 77mg; Dietary fiber 5g;
Calories from fat 10%

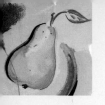

1 teaspoon margarine

1 large onion, chopped

2 celery stalks, chopped

5 cups (40 fl oz/1.25 l) Chicken Stock (recipe on page 206) or reduced sodium chicken broth

1½ lb (750 g) potatoes, cut into 1-inch (2.5-cm) cubes

¼ cup (⅓ oz/10 g) chopped fresh parsley

¼ cup (1 oz/30 g) grated lowfat cheddar cheese

¼ teaspoon ground white pepper

4 fresh flat-leaf (Italian) parsley sprigs

Shopping Tip

✳ If fresh herbs are not available, substitute dried herbs, which have a stronger flavor. Use a ratio of 1:4, that is, about one-fourth of the amount of dried herbs to the fresh herbs called for in a recipe.

Potato Soup

Preparation: 25 minutes ✳ *Cooking: 55 minutes* ✳ *Serves 4*

Leaving the potato skins intact adds extra texture, vitamins and fiber to this puréed soup, which has the look of a traditional cream soup but only a fraction of the fat of dairy products.

✳ In a large saucepan over medium heat, melt the margarine. Add the onion and celery and sauté, stirring frequently, until tender, about 10 minutes.

✳ Add the stock or broth and potatoes, increase the heat to medium-high and bring to a boil.

✳ Reduce the heat to low, cover and simmer until the potatoes are tender when pierced with a fork, about 30 minutes.

✳ Remove from the heat, add the chopped parsley, stir to mix well and let stand for 5 minutes.

✳ Strain the soup, reserving the liquid, and transfer the vegetables to a food processor with the metal blade or to a blender. Add 1 cup (8 fl oz/250 ml) of the reserved liquid to the vegetable mixture and process until smooth.

✳ In the same saucepan over medium-low heat, combine the purée, remaining reserved liquid, cheese and pepper. Simmer, stirring frequently, until the cheese melts, about 5 minutes.

✳ To serve, divide among 4 individual bowls. Top each with a parsley sprig.

Nutritional Analysis per Serving

Calories 207 (Kilojoules 868); Total fat 2g; Saturated fat 0g; Protein 8g; Cholesterol 1mg; Carbohydrates 37g; Sodium 841mg; Dietary fiber 4g; Calories from fat 8%

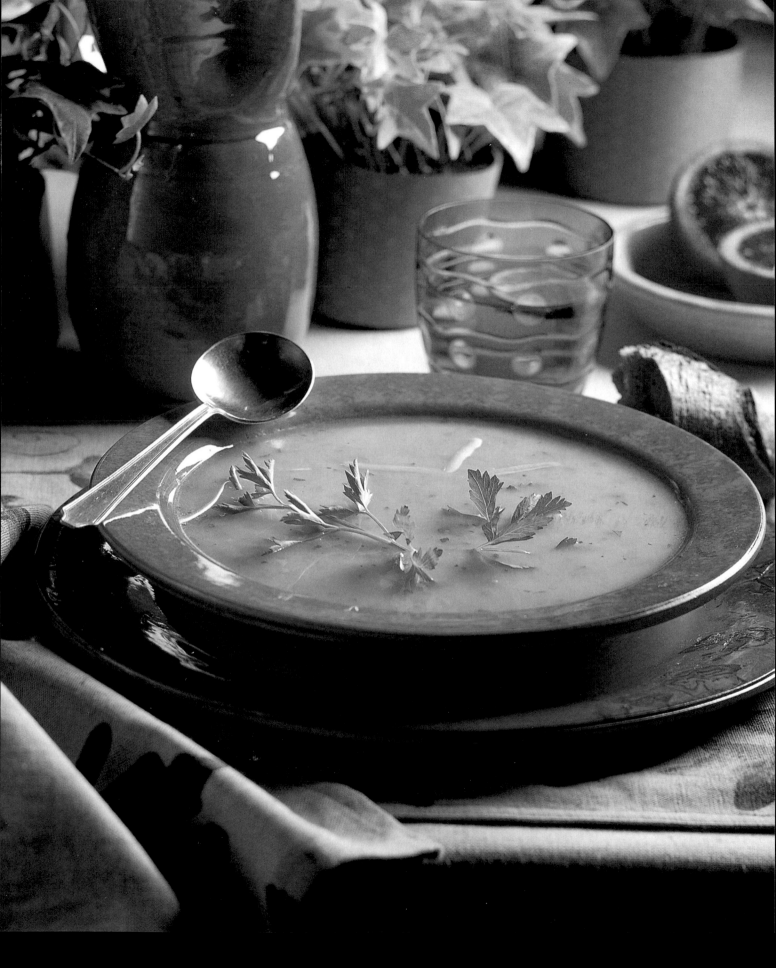

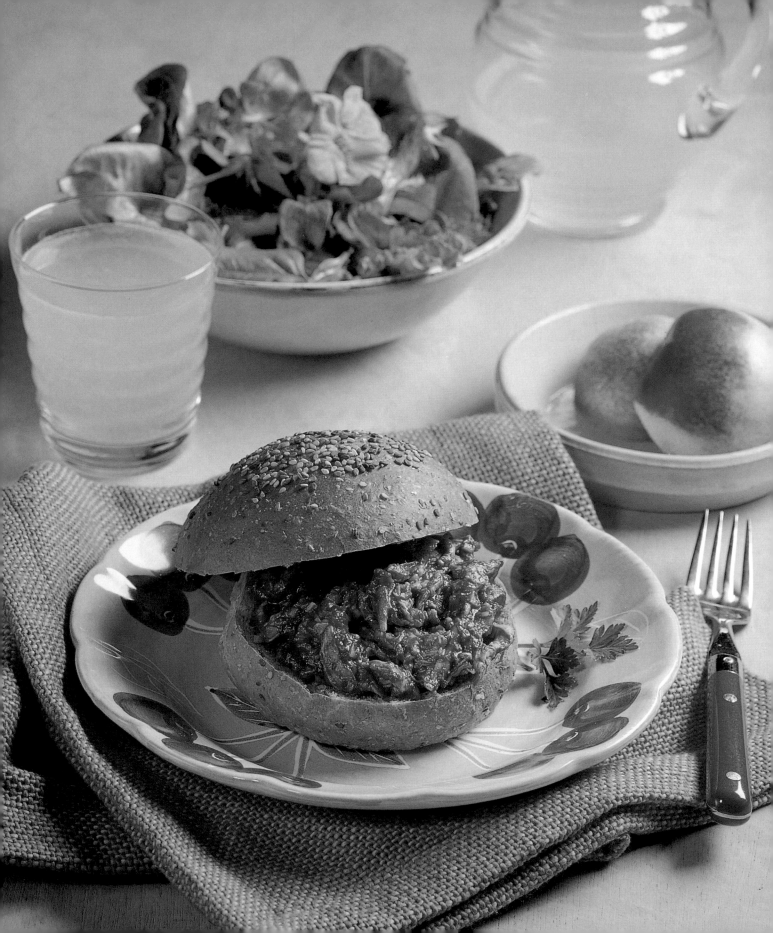

Shredded Chicken Sandwich

1 lb (500 g) skinless, boneless chicken breast, cut into thin strips

3 garlic cloves, peeled and minced

1 cup (8 fl oz/250 ml) canned tomato purée

¼ cup (2 fl oz/60 ml) dark molasses

2 tablespoons Dijon-style mustard

2 tablespoons white wine vinegar

1 teaspoon chili powder

¼ teaspoon salt

¼ teaspoon hot pepper sauce

4 whole wheat (wholemeal) rolls, halved and toasted

Storage Tip

✳ The shredded chicken with its spicy sauce can be stored in an airtight container in the refrigerator for up to 4 days.

Preparation: 10 minutes ✳ *Cooking: 20 minutes* ✳ *Serves 4*

In just 30 minutes, you can enjoy the flavors of slow-cooked Southern barbecue—tomatoes, molasses, mustard, vinegar, chili powder and hot pepper sauce—in this deliciously healthy, traditionally messy sandwich.

✳ Coat a large nonstick frying pan with nonstick cooking spray and place over medium heat. Add the chicken and sauté until it is no longer pink in the center, about 5 minutes.

✳ To make the sauce, in a medium bowl, combine the garlic, tomato purée, molasses, mustard, vinegar, chili powder, salt and hot pepper sauce and whisk until blended.

✳ When the chicken is cooked, add the sauce, bring to a boil, reduce the heat to low and simmer until the liquid is reduced by half and the chicken is tender, about 10 minutes. Using a slotted spoon, transfer the chicken to a work surface. Using 2 forks, pull the chicken into thin shreds and return it to the sauce.

✳ To serve, place one half of each bun on 4 individual plates. Top each with an equal amount of the chicken, sauce and the other half of the bun.

Nutritional Analysis per Serving

Calories 354 (Kilojoules 1,486); Total fat 4g; Saturated fat 1g; Protein 33g; Cholesterol 66mg; Carbohydrates 46g; Sodium 963mg; Dietary fiber 6g; Calories from fat 11%

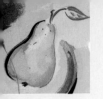

1 lb (500 g) ground chicken breast

½ cup (1½ oz/45 g) chopped green
(spring) onions, green and
white parts

¼ cup (1 oz/30 g) dried bread crumbs

2 teaspoons Worcestershire sauce

½ teaspoon hot pepper sauce

¼ teaspoon salt

1 egg white

4 whole wheat (wholemeal)
hamburger buns, halved and
lightly toasted

4 lettuce leaves

Creamy Horseradish

1 cup (8 oz/250 g) nonfat dairy
sour cream

¼ cup (2 oz/60 g) drained, grated
horseradish

2 tablespoons white wine vinegar

¼ teaspoon ground black pepper

Shopping Tip

✳ When buying ground chicken, be sure
that it is all lowfat breast meat. You can
easily grind your own meat by purchasing
skinless, boneless chicken breasts, cutting
them into chunks and chopping them in
a food processor with a metal blade.

Spicy Chicken Burgers
with Creamy Horseradish

Preparation: 15 minutes ✳ Cooking: 10 minutes ✳ Serves 4

*Hot sauce, green onions and a horseradish dressing spice up the flavor
of these healthy burgers. Make the Creamy Horseradish before you cook
your burgers.*

✳ In a large bowl, combine the chicken, green onions, bread
crumbs, Worcestershire sauce, hot pepper sauce, salt and egg
white. Stir to mix well. Transfer to a work surface, divide into
4 equal portions and shape each portion into a patty 1 inch
(2.5 cm) thick.

✳ Coat a large nonstick frying pan with nonstick cooking spray.
Place the frying pan over medium heat, add the patties and cook,
covered, until browned, about 5 minutes. Turn and cook, covered,
until the chicken is no longer pink in the center, about 5 minutes.

✳ To serve, spread 1 tablespoon of the Creamy Horseradish on
each half bun. Place one half of each bun on 4 individual plates.
Top each with a lettuce leaf, a burger and the other half of the bun.

Creamy Horseradish

✳ In a small bowl, combine the sour cream, horseradish, vinegar
and pepper and whisk until blended.

✳ Store in an airtight container in the refrigerator for up to
3 days. One serving is 2 tablespoons.

Nutritional Analysis per Serving

Calories 279 (Kilojoules 1,174); Total fat 4g; Saturated fat 1g; Protein 34g;
Cholesterol 66mg; Carbohydrates 26g; Sodium 542mg; Dietary fiber 3g;
Calories from fat 13%

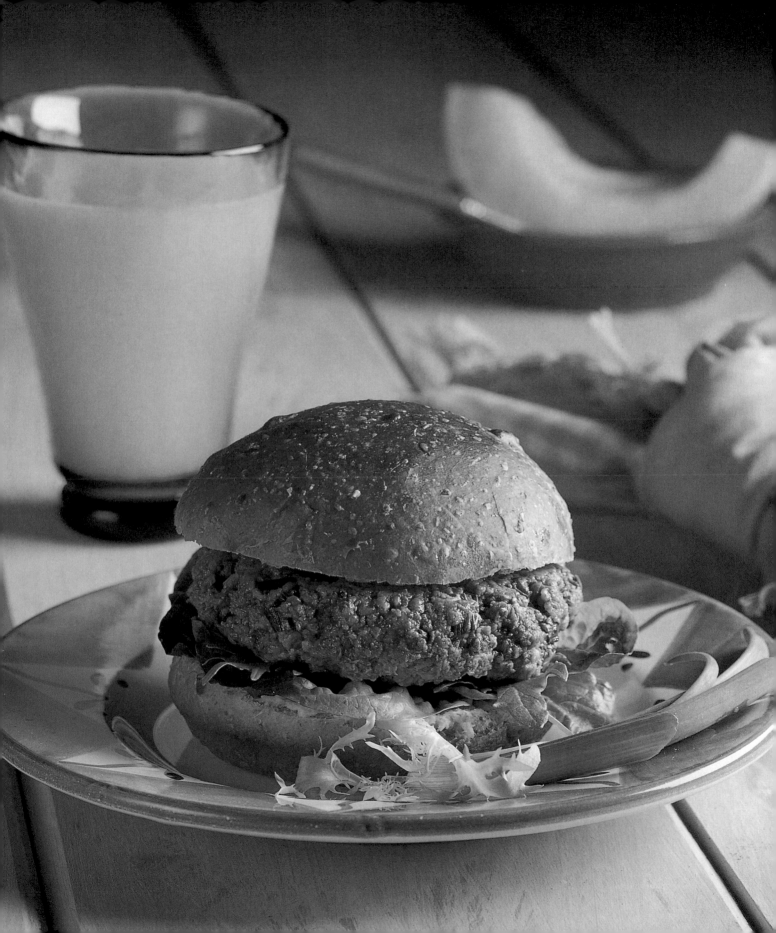

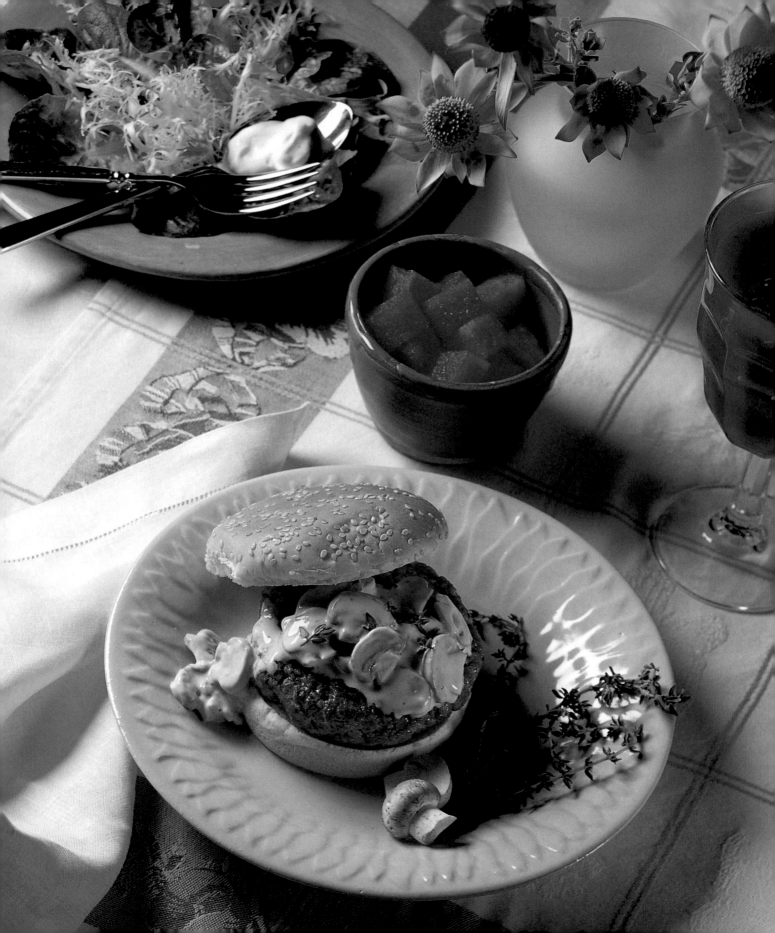

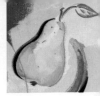

1 lb (500 g) ground turkey breast

1 small onion, chopped

¼ cup (1 oz/30 g) dried bread crumbs

1 egg white

¼ teaspoon salt

¼ teaspoon ground mustard

½ teaspoon ground black pepper

4 oz (125 g) fresh mushrooms, sliced

½ cup (4 fl oz/125 ml) Chicken Stock
(recipe on page 206) or reduced
sodium chicken broth

1 tablespoon chopped fresh thyme

½ cup (4 oz/125 g) nonfat dairy
sour cream

4 sesame seed hamburger buns, halved

Turkey Burgers with Mushroom Sauce

Preparation: 15 minutes ✳ Cooking: 15 minutes ✳ Serves 4

Readily available ground turkey breast has a robust flavor and is a lowfat alternative to ground beef. When shopping, look for ground turkey breast. It is lower in calories and fat than regular ground turkey meat, which often has the dark meat and the turkey skin ground with the breast meat. You can also grind your own turkey breast using a food processor.

✳ In a large bowl, combine the turkey, onion, bread crumbs, egg white, salt, mustard and ¼ teaspoon of the pepper and toss to mix well. Transfer to a work surface, divide into 4 equal portions and shape each portion into a patty 1 inch (2.5 cm) thick.

✳ Coat a large nonstick frying pan with nonstick cooking spray. Place the frying pan over medium heat, add the patties and cook, covered, until browned, about 5 minutes. Turn and cook, covered, until the turkey is no longer pink in the center, about 5 minutes.

✳ To make the mushroom sauce, coat a small nonstick frying pan with nonstick cooking spray. Place the frying pan over medium heat, add the mushrooms and sauté until they are tender and release their juices, about 3 minutes. Add the stock or broth and thyme, bring to a boil, reduce the heat to low and simmer for 5 minutes. Add the sour cream and remaining ¼ teaspoon pepper and simmer until the sauce thickens, about 2 minutes.

✳ To serve, place one half of each bun on 4 individual plates. Top with a burger, an equal amount of the mushroom sauce and the other half of the bun.

Nutritional Analysis per Serving

Calories 330 (Kilojoules 1,384); Total fat 4g; Saturated fat 1g; Protein 37g; Cholesterol 70mg; Carbohydrates 33g; Sodium 543mg; Dietary fiber 2g; Calories from fat 13%

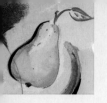

12 oz (375 g) water-packed albacore
tuna, drained

1 red bell pepper (capsicum), seeded,
deribbed and diced

½ cup (4 oz/125 g) nonfat plain yogurt

2 tablespoons chopped fresh flat-leaf
(Italian) parsley

1 tablespoon Dijon-style mustard

1 tablespoon red wine vinegar

¼ teaspoon ground black pepper

3 oz (90 g) arugula (rocket), stems
trimmed

2 whole wheat (wholemeal) pita
breads, 8 inches (20 cm) in
diameter, halved

Nutrition Tip

✳ Check those tuna cans carefully before
purchase. The nutritional differences
between oil-packed chunk light tuna and
water-packed solid white are remarkable.
Per 3 oz (90 g) serving, oil-packed contains
165 calories, 7 g fat, 1.4 g saturated fat
and 24 g protein. In comparison, the same
amount of water-packed contains just
135 calories, 1 g fat and .3 g saturated fat,
as well as 33 g protein.

Tuna Salad Sandwich

Preparation: 25 minutes ✳ Serves 4

*The combination of tangy yogurt and mustard, peppery arugula and
vitamin C-rich red bell pepper makes for a refreshing change of pace from
everyday tuna sandwiches.*

✳ In a large bowl, combine the tuna and bell pepper and toss
to mix well. Add the yogurt, parsley, mustard, vinegar and pepper
and stir until blended.

✳ To serve, place an equal amount of the tuna mixture and arugula
into each pita half. One serving is a half pita.

Nutritional Analysis per Serving

Calories 249 (Kilojoules 1,046); Total fat 3g; Saturated fat 1g; Protein 28g;
Cholesterol 34mg; Carbohydrates 27g; Sodium 658mg; Dietary fiber 4g;
Calories from fat 11%

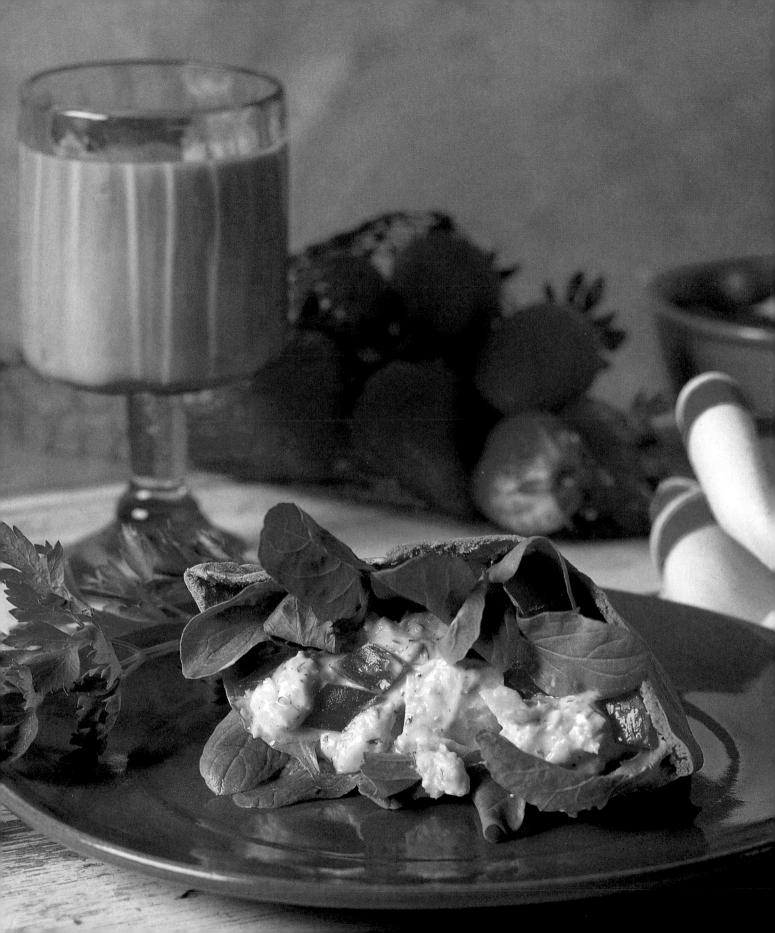

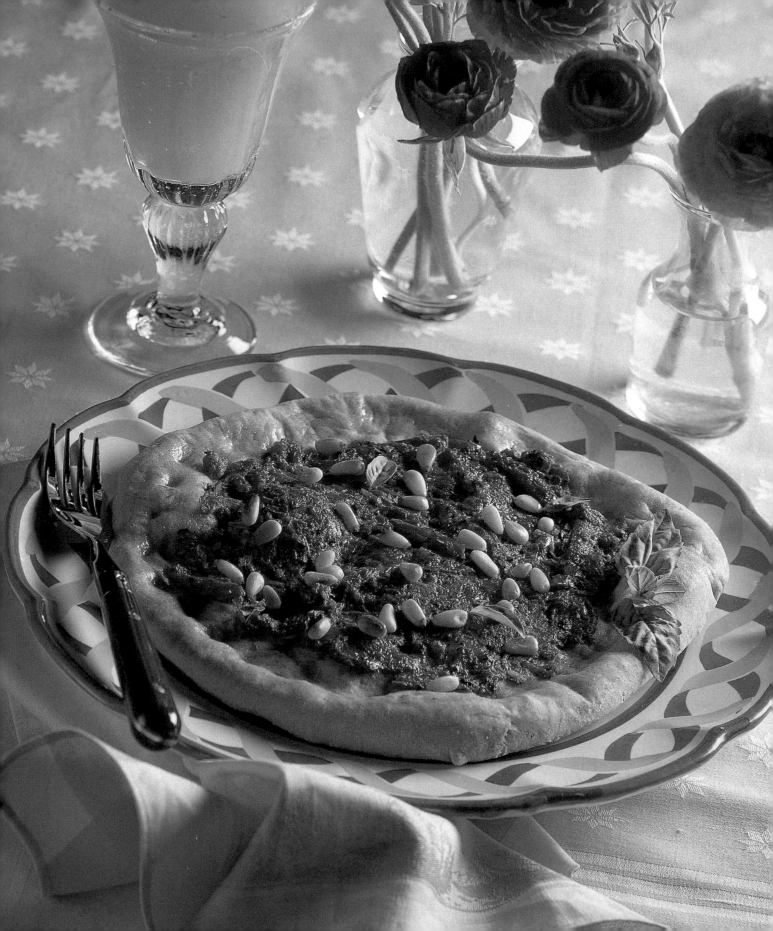

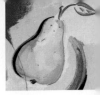

Tomato-Basil Pizza

Preparation: 25 minutes ✳ Cooking: 20 minutes ✳ Serves 4

Tomatoes and basil are a traditional Mediterranean flavor combination that is well represented in this quick pizza. In the summer, try using different types of fresh tomatoes, including red or yellow cherry tomatoes. When pressed for time, spread the sauce on commercial pizza bread shells and bake as directed on the package.

30 sun-dried tomatoes, packed without oil

1 lb (500 g) plum (Roma) tomatoes, peeled, seeded and diced

½ cup (4 fl oz/125 ml) Chicken Stock (recipe on page 206) or reduced sodium chicken broth

½ cup (½ oz/15 g) firmly packed fresh basil leaves

2 garlic cloves, peeled and minced

3 tablespoons grated Romano cheese

¼ teaspoon salt

¼ teaspoon ground black pepper

1 teaspoon olive oil

1 lb (500 g) Karen's Pizza Dough (recipe on page 185)

2 tablespoons pine nuts, lightly toasted

✳ Preheat an oven to 450°F (230°C). Coat 2 large baking sheets with nonstick cooking spray.

✳ In a small saucepan over medium heat, combine the sun-dried tomatoes, fresh tomatoes and stock or broth. Bring to a boil, reduce the heat to low and simmer until the sun-dried tomatoes are tender, about 5 minutes.

✳ In a food processor with the metal blade or in a blender, combine the basil, garlic, Romano cheese, salt and pepper. Process until smooth. With the motor running, gradually add the olive oil and process until blended. Add the tomato mixture to the basil mixture and pulse on and off until just blended.

✳ Divide the pizza dough into 4 equal portions. On a lightly floured work surface, roll out each portion into an 8-inch (20-cm) round. Place on the prepared sheets and form a ½-inch (12-mm) raised lip around the edges. Top each round with an equal amount of the tomato and basil mixture and pine nuts, leaving a ½-inch (12-mm) border around the edges.

✳ Bake until the crusts are golden, about 15 minutes.

✳ To serve, place on 4 individual plates.

Cooking Tip

✳ To peel fresh tomatoes, bring a saucepan of water to a boil. With a small, sharp knife, cut out the core at the stem end of each tomato and score a shallow X in the skin at the opposite end. One at a time and using a slotted spoon, immerse the tomatoes in the boiling water for about 10 seconds to loosen their skins. Lift out and dip in a bowl of cold water to cool. Then, starting at the X, peel off the skin, using the knife blade to help you if necessary.

Nutritional Analysis per Serving

Calories 618 (Kilojoules 2,596); Total fat 14g; Saturated fat 2g; Protein 23g; Cholesterol 4mg; Carbohydrates 106g; Sodium 835mg; Dietary fiber 14g; Calories from fat 20%

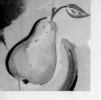

½ cup (½ oz/15 g) dried porcini
  mushrooms, stemmed
½ cup (½ oz/15 g) dried shiitake
  mushrooms, stemmed
1 cup (8 fl oz/250 ml) Chicken Stock
  (recipe on page 206) or reduced
  sodium chicken broth
2 tablespoons chopped fresh thyme
¼ teaspoon ground black pepper
1 lb (500 g) Karen's Pizza Dough
  (recipe on page 185)
2 teaspoons extra-virgin olive oil
¼ cup (1 oz/30 g) grated Romano
  cheese
2 tablespoons chopped fresh flat-leaf
  (Italian) parsley

Shopping Tip

❋ Well-stocked markets carry both of
these dried mushrooms. You may also find
porcini mushrooms in Italian delicatessens
and shiitake mushrooms in Asian markets.

Mushroom-Cheese Pizza

Preparation: 25 minutes ❋ Cooking: 25 minutes ❋ Serves 4

*Two types of dried mushrooms give a wonderful, earthy flavor to this
foccacia-style pizza—that is, a pizza without sauce as a topping. Unlike
many pizzas, which are just as good hot or cold, this one is best eaten
soon after baking as it tends to dry out as it cools.*

❋ Preheat an oven to 450°F (230°C). Coat a large baking sheet
with nonstick cooking spray.

❋ In a small saucepan over medium heat, combine the mushrooms, stock or broth and thyme. Bring to a boil, reduce the heat
to low and simmer until the liquid is absorbed, about 15 minutes.
Add the pepper and stir to mix well. Cool the mushrooms in the
pan, then transfer to a work surface and slice into thin strips.

❋ On a lightly floured work surface, roll out the pizza dough
into a 12-inch (30-cm) round. Place on the prepared sheet and
form a ½-inch (12-mm) raised lip around the edge. Brush the
olive oil over the dough. Top with the mushrooms and Romano
cheese, leaving a ½-inch (12-mm) border around the edge.

❋ Bake until the crust is golden, about 15 minutes.

❋ To serve, top the pizza with the parsley. Slice into quarters
and place on 4 individual plates.

Nutritional Analysis per Serving

Calories 542 (Kilojoules 2,277); Total fat 13g; Saturated fat 1g; Protein 19g;
Cholesterol 7mg; Carbohydrates 89g; Sodium 783mg; Dietary fiber 11g;
Calories from fat 22%

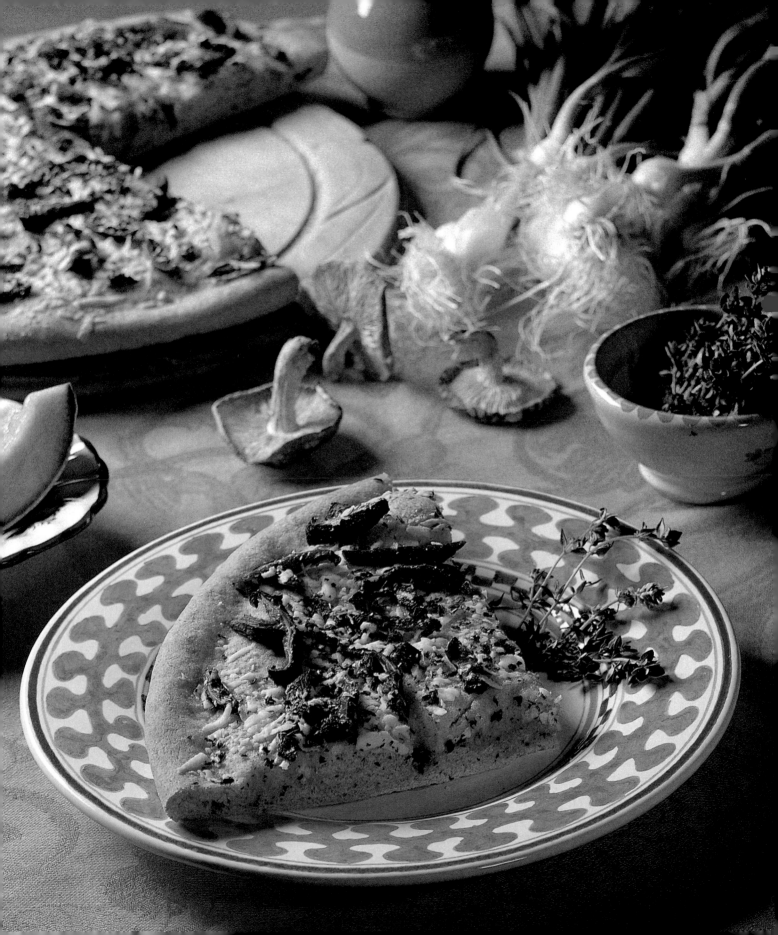

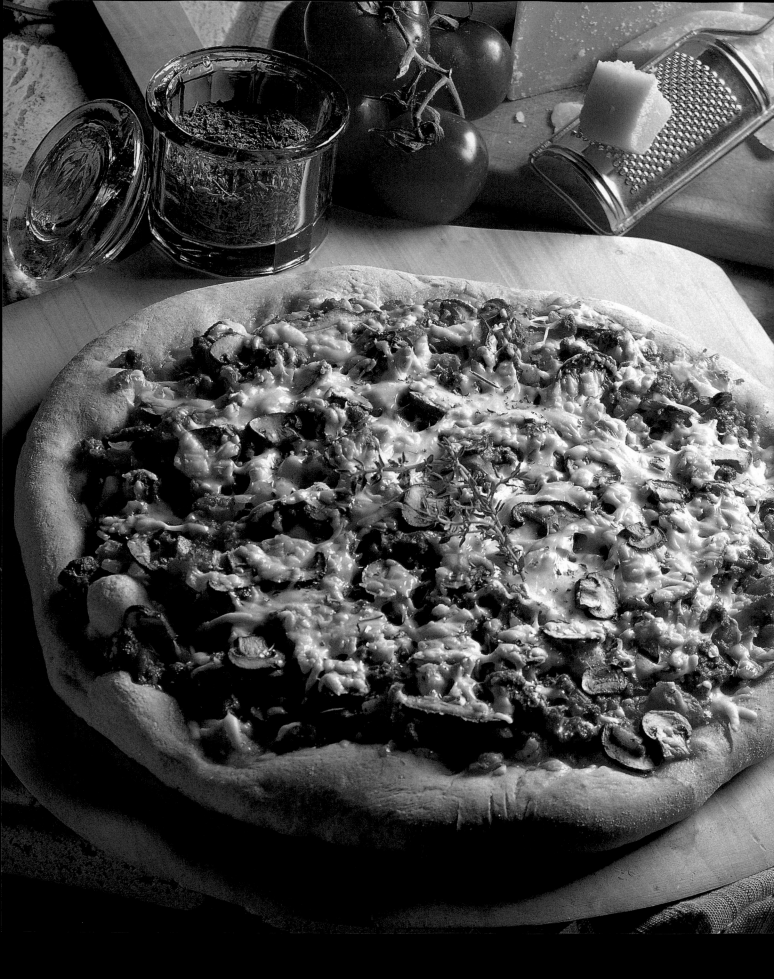

1 onion, chopped

2 garlic cloves, peeled and minced

8 oz (250 g) ground bison or lean
(10%) ground beef

1 tablespoon herbes de Provence

8 oz (250 g) fresh mushrooms, sliced

2 lb (1 kg) plum (Roma) tomatoes,
peeled, seeded and diced

1 teaspoon salt

½ teaspoon ground black pepper

¼ cup (1 oz/30 g) grated Parmesan
cheese

1 lb (500 g) Karen's Pizza Dough
(recipe on page 185)

1 cup (4 oz/125 g) shredded lowfat
mozzarella cheese

Cooking Tip

✳ Herbes de Provence are a blend of
dried herbs typical of Provence, France.
To make your own, combine ½ teaspoon
each of thyme, rosemary, sage, marjoram,
basil, fennel seed and mint.

Ted's Favorite Pizza

Preparation: 25 minutes ✳ Cooking: 25 minutes ✳ Serves 4

*Ted enjoys this pizza because it features bison, which we raise on our
ranch in Montana. The metabolism of bison is such that fat is not deposited
within the muscles, resulting in a much leaner red meat than beef. Because
of its health benefits and great taste, bison meat is growing in popularity.
If bison is not yet available in your store, check the Resources Guide on
page 240 for mail-order sources. You may find it becomes your favorite
pizza topping, too.*

✳ Preheat an oven to 425°F (220°C). Coat a large baking sheet
with nonstick cooking spray.

✳ Coat a large nonstick frying pan with nonstick cooking spray.
Place over medium heat, add the onion and garlic and sauté for
2 minutes. Add the bison or beef and herbs and sauté until the
meat is no longer pink, about 5 minutes for bison and 7 minutes
for beef. Add the mushrooms, tomatoes, salt and pepper and
simmer until the liquid evaporates, about 10 minutes. Remove
from the heat and stir in the Parmesan cheese.

✳ On a lightly floured work surface, roll out the pizza dough
into a 12-inch (30-cm) round. Place on the prepared sheet and
form a ½-inch (12-mm) raised lip around the edge. Top with the
meat mixture and the mozzarella, leaving a ½-inch (12-mm)
border around the edge.

✳ Bake until the crust is golden and the cheese is bubbly, about
15 minutes.

✳ To serve, slice into quarters and place on 4 individual plates.

Nutritional Analysis per Serving

Calories 696 (Kilojoules 2,923); Total fat 16g; Saturated fat 5g; Protein 41g;
Cholesterol 51mg; Carbohydrates 101g; Sodium 1,432mg; Dietary fiber 14g;
Calories from fat 20%

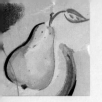

1 teaspoon plus 1 tablespoon olive oil

2 garlic cloves, peeled and minced

2 tablespoons chopped fresh oregano

½ teaspoon salt

½ teaspoon ground black pepper

¾ lb (375 g) lean beef tenderloin, trimmed of visible fat and cut into 1-inch (2.5-cm) chunks

1 cucumber (about 12 oz/375 g), seeded and chopped

2 plum (Roma) tomatoes (6 oz/185 g), sliced

1 small red onion, thinly sliced

¼ cup (1 oz/30 g) crumbled feta cheese

¼ cup (⅓ oz/10 g) chopped fresh flat-leaf (Italian) parsley

4 Kalamata olives, pitted

2 tablespoons lemon juice

1 teaspoon finely grated lemon zest

Cooking Tip

✳ To pit an olive, use an olive pitter, which grips the olive and pushes out the pit. Or, using a small, sharp knife, slit the olive lengthwise down to the pit and pry away the flesh.

Greek Salad

Preparation: 20 minutes ✳ *Cooking: 5 minutes* ✳ *Serves 4*

In addition to the preparation time, the beef must marinate for 1 hour. While you can use any type of olive in this dish, Kalamata olives provide the authentic taste of Greece, evoking warm days spent on island beaches. For this reason, the salad is ideal to serve when lunching outdoors.

✳ In a glass baking dish, combine the 1 teaspoon olive oil and half the garlic, oregano, salt and pepper and stir to mix well. Add the beef and toss to coat. Cover and refrigerate to marinate for 1 hour.

✳ Coat a frying pan with nonstick cooking spray and place over medium-high heat. Using a slotted spoon, transfer the beef to the pan, reserving the marinade, and cook, stirring frequently, for 3 minutes. Add the marinade to the pan and cook until the beef is no longer pink in the center, about 2 minutes more.

✳ Using a slotted spoon, transfer the beef to a large bowl. Discard the marinade. To the bowl, add the cucumber, tomatoes, onion, cheese, parsley and olives.

✳ In a small bowl, combine the 1 tablespoon olive oil, garlic, oregano, salt and pepper and the lemon juice and lemon zest, and whisk until blended. Add to the vegetable mixture and toss to coat well.

✳ To serve, divide among 4 individual plates.

Nutritional Analysis per Serving

Calories 250 (Kilojoules 1,051); Total fat 15g; Saturated fat 4g; Protein 20g; Cholesterol 59mg; Carbohydrates 10g; Sodium 500mg; Dietary fiber 2g; Calories from fat 52%

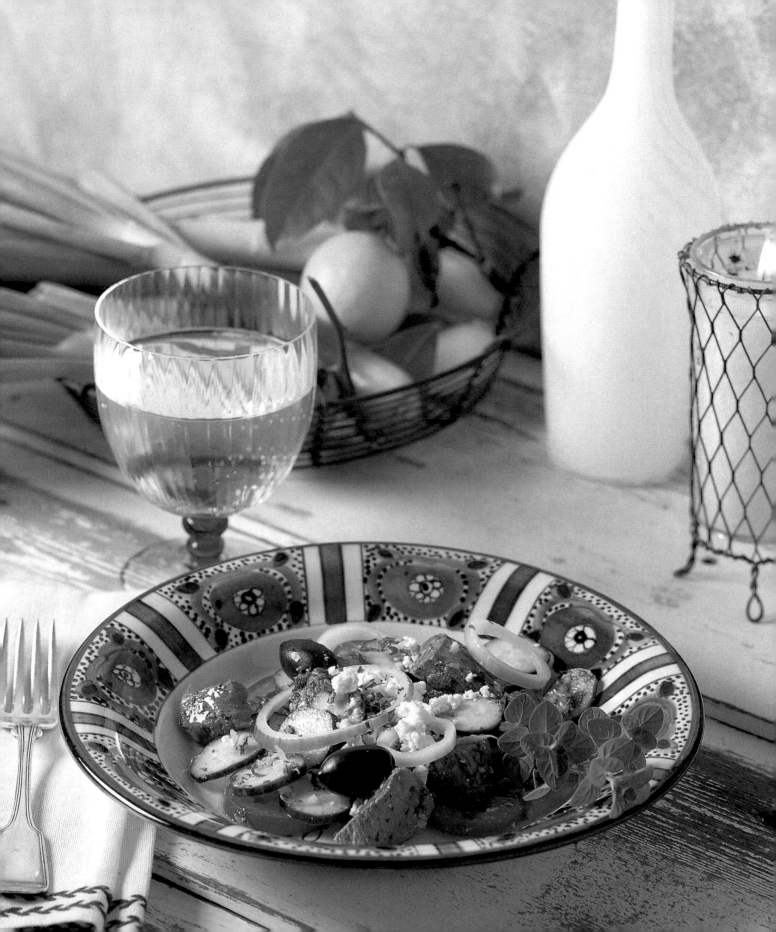

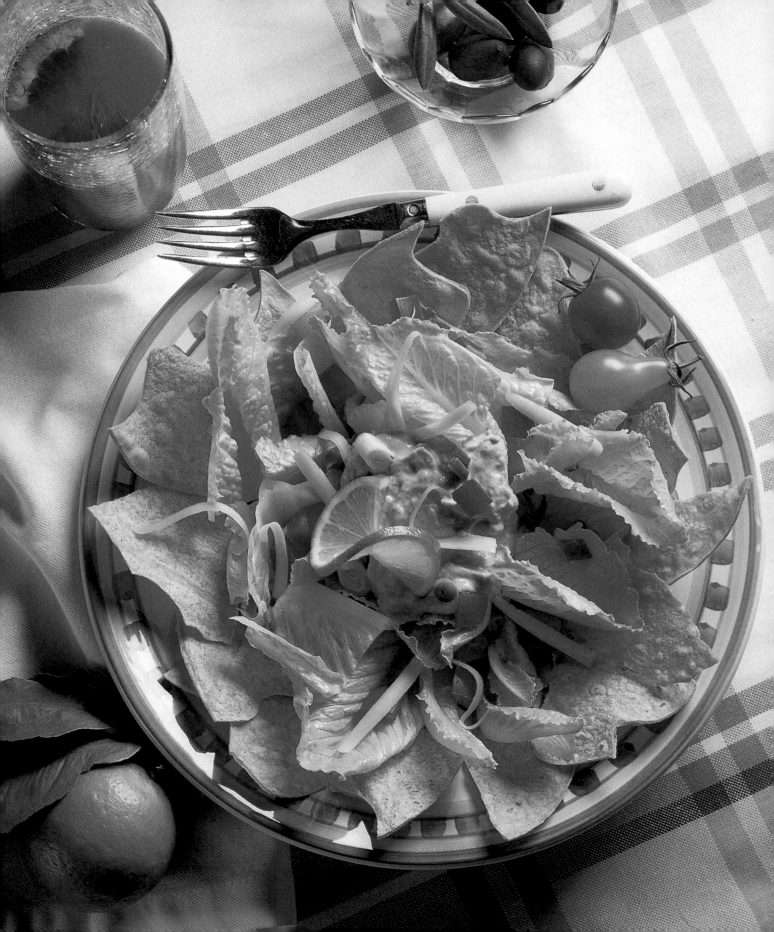

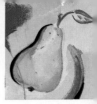

8 corn tortillas, 8 inches (20 cm) in diameter

4 cups (12 oz/375 g) chopped romaine (cos) lettuce

3 plum (Roma) tomatoes, seeded and chopped

1 green (spring) onion, green and white parts, chopped

¼ cup (1 oz/30 g) grated lowfat cheddar cheese

Avocado Dressing

1 avocado, peeled, pitted and mashed

½ cup (4 oz/125 g) nonfat dairy sour cream

2 tablespoons lime juice

1 garlic clove, peeled and minced

½ teaspoon chili powder

Storage Tip

✳ The Avocado Dressing can be stored in an airtight container in the refrigerator for up to 4 days.

Taco Salad with Avocado Dressing

Preparation: 25 minutes ✳ Cooking: 15 minutes ✳ Serves 4

Avocados are a wonderful fruit but they do contain fat and should be used sparingly. This recipe uses just 1 avocado for 4 servings, which will not detrimentally affect your nutritional goals. Seek out Hass avocados with thick dark pebbly skins as they are considered to have the best flavor and texture. Make sure the avocado is absolutely ripe for optimum taste. For a healthy snack, skip the salad and serve the homemade chips with the dressing as a dip.

✳ Preheat an oven to 425°F (220°C).

✳ To make the chips, place the tortillas on ungreased baking sheets and bake until crisp, about 15 minutes, turning halfway through the cooking time. Cool to the touch and break into 2-inch (5-cm) pieces.

✳ In a large bowl, combine the lettuce, tomatoes, green onion and cheese and toss to mix well.

✳ To serve, line 4 individual salad plates with an equal amount of the chips. Top each with an equal amount of the salad mixture and Avocado Dressing.

Avocado Dressing

✳ In a food processor with the metal blade or in a blender, combine the avocado, sour cream, lime juice, garlic and chili powder. Process until smooth. One serving is 3 tablespoons.

Nutritional Analysis per Serving

Calories 249 (Kilojoules 1,046); Total fat 10g; Saturated fat 1g; Protein 9g; Cholesterol 1mg; Carbohydrates 34g; Sodium 220mg; Dietary fiber 6g; Calories from fat 34%

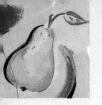

Lentil and Smoked Turkey Salad

Preparation: 20 minutes ✳ *Cooking: 15 minutes* ✳ *Serves 4*

5 cups (40 fl oz/1.25 l) water

1½ cups (10½ oz/330 g) dried lentils, rinsed and picked over to remove stones

1 small red onion, chopped

1 tablespoon chopped fresh thyme

½ teaspoon ground allspice

¼ cup (2 fl oz/60 ml) red wine vinegar

1 tablespoon Dijon-style mustard

1½ tablespoons olive oil

2 celery stalks, chopped

2 carrots, chopped

¼ cup (⅓ oz/10 g) chopped fresh flat-leaf (Italian) parsley

1 teaspoon salt

¼ teaspoon ground black pepper

6 oz (185 g) smoked turkey breast, cut into bite-sized pieces

Lentils, the disk-shaped seeds of a legume plant native to Asia, are an excellent source of nonfat protein in a healthy diet. Several different colors of lentils are available, and they are interchangeable for this cold salad. Smoked turkey is available in the delicatessen section of supermarkets.

✳ In a medium saucepan over medium-high heat, combine the water, lentils, onion, thyme and allspice. Bring to a boil, reduce the heat to low and simmer until the lentils are tender but still intact, about 15 minutes.

✳ Drain the lentil mixture and transfer to a large bowl. Add the vinegar, mustard, olive oil, celery, carrots, parsley, salt and pepper. Refrigerate the salad for at least 15 minutes to allow the lentils and vegetables to marinate in the dressing, then bring to room temperature.

✳ To serve, divide among 4 individual plates. Top each with an equal amount of the turkey pieces.

Nutritional Analysis per Serving

Calories 385 (Kilojoules 1,616); Total fat 7g; Saturated fat 1g; Protein 31g; Cholesterol 18mg; Carbohydrates 51g; Sodium 1,081mg; Dietary fiber 11g; Calories from fat 17%

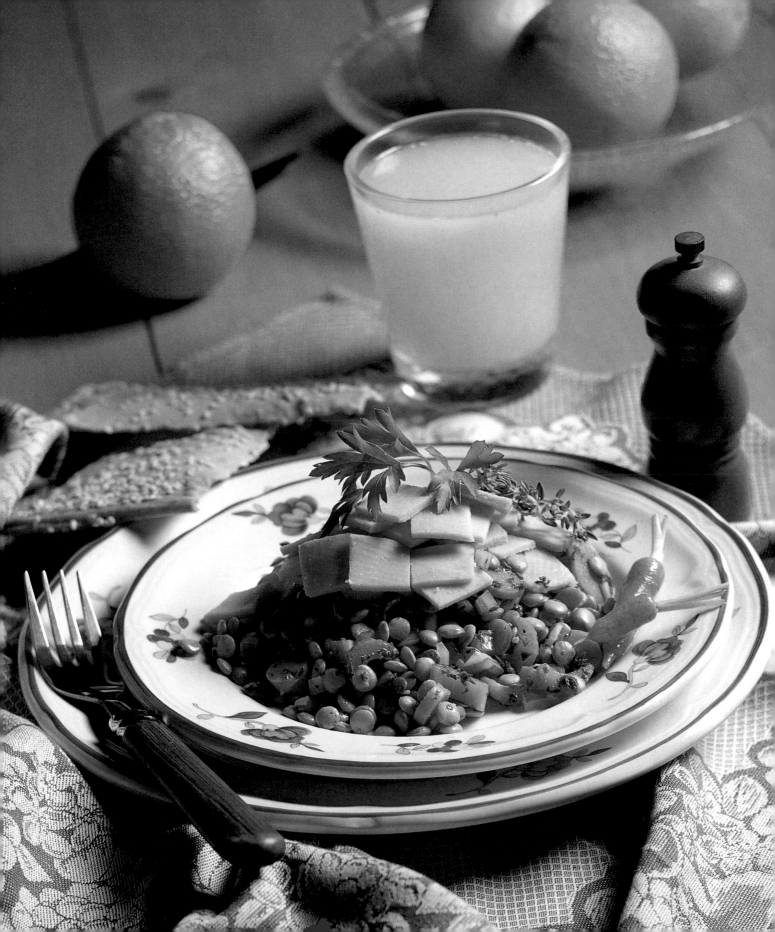

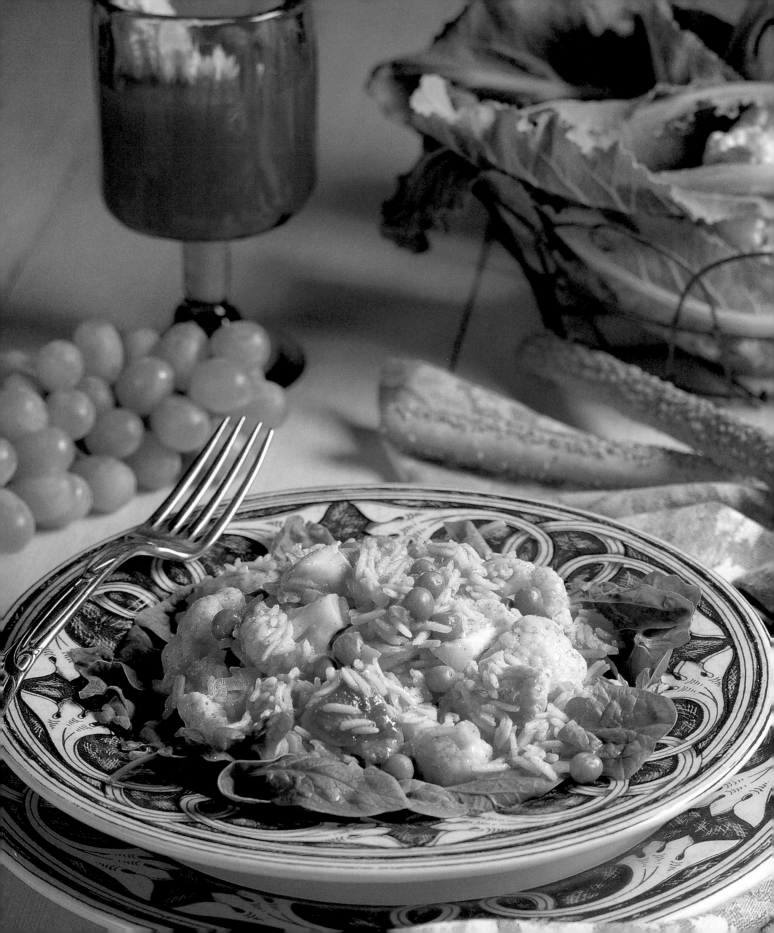

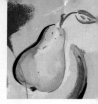

Curried Chicken, Rice and Spinach Salad

2 teaspoons dark sesame oil

2 shallots, peeled and minced

2 garlic cloves, peeled and minced

1 lb (500 g) skinless, boneless chicken breast, cut into 1-inch (2.5-cm) cubes

3 cups (24 fl oz/750 ml) Chicken Stock (recipe on page 206) or reduced sodium chicken broth

2 teaspoons curry powder

1 teaspoon ground cumin

⅔ cup (5 oz/155 g) basmati rice

½ teaspoon salt

¼ teaspoon ground black pepper

2 cups (10 oz/315 g) green peas

2 cups (4 oz/125 g) cauliflower florets

2 cups (14 oz/440 g) chopped spinach

Cooking Tip

✱ To peel and mince garlic cloves, separate them as needed from the whole head of garlic. Place the clove on a steady work surface. Cover it with the side of the blade of a large knife. Keeping the knife's cutting edge safely clear of your hand, press down firmly but carefully on the side of the blade to crush the clove slightly; the skin will slip off easily. Then, thinly slice the clove lengthwise; cut the slices lengthwise into thin strips; and cut finely across the strips to mince them.

Preparation: 25 minutes ✱ Cooking: 50 minutes ✱ Serves 4

Warm salads like this one are a good choice for lunch on a crisp spring afternoon. The flavors of India are represented here. Curry is a generic term for spice blends common to the Indian subcontinent, including cumin, chili powder and turmeric. Basmati is an aromatic long-grain Indian rice.

✱ In a large nonstick frying pan over medium heat, heat the oil. Add the shallots and garlic and sauté until tender, about 2 minutes. Add the chicken and sauté until browned and no longer pink in the center, about 5 minutes.

✱ Add the stock or broth, curry and cumin and bring to a boil.

✱ Add the rice, salt and pepper, reduce the heat to low and simmer for 20 minutes.

✱ Add the peas and cauliflower and simmer until the rice is soft, about 20 minutes more.

✱ To serve, divide the spinach among 4 individual plates. Top each with an equal amount of the rice mixture.

Nutritional Analysis per Serving

Calories 383 (Kilojoules 1,608); Total fat 6g; Saturated fat 1g; Protein 40g; Cholesterol 66mg; Carbohydrates 46g; Sodium 874mg; Dietary fiber 7g; Calories from fat 13%

8 cups (64 fl oz/2 l) water

10 sun-dried tomatoes, packed
without oil

8 oz (250 g) dried orzo

¾ lb (12 oz/375 g) shelled green peas

¼ cup (½ oz/15 g) chopped fresh basil

¼ cup (½ oz/15 g) chopped fresh
flat-leaf (Italian) parsley

3 tablespoons balsamic vinegar

1 tablespoon olive oil

¼ teaspoon salt

¼ teaspoon ground black pepper

2 tablespoons grated Romano cheese

Shopping Tip

* Green peas are in season from spring
through summer. At other times of the
year, substitute frozen peas, thawed.

Orzo, Sun-Dried Tomato and Pea Salad

*Preparation: 15 minutes * Cooking: 10 minutes * Serves 4*

*Orzo, a cut of pasta resembling grains of rice, gives an interesting texture
to this dish. If you don't have orzo, substitute any small dried pasta
shape. Sun-dried tomatoes bring a flash of summer flavor to a salad that
can be made year round.*

* In a small saucepan over high heat, combine 1 cup (8 fl oz/
250 ml) of the water and the tomatoes. Bring to a boil, reduce
the heat to low and simmer until the tomatoes are tender, about
15 minutes. Drain, reserving the liquid, and slice the tomatoes
into thin strips.

* In a large pot over high heat, bring 6 cups (48 fl oz/1.5 l)
water to a boil. Add the orzo and cook according to the package
directions, about 10 minutes. Drain, rinse in cold water, drain
again and place in a large bowl.

* In a medium saucepan over high heat, bring the remaining
water to a boil. Add the peas, reduce the heat to low and simmer,
covered, until the peas are tender-crisp, about 5 minutes. Drain,
rinse in cold water, drain again and add to the orzo.

* In a small bowl, combine the reserved liquid, basil, parsley,
vinegar, oil, salt and pepper and whisk until blended. Add to
the bowl with the orzo. Add the tomatoes, peas and cheese. Toss
to coat well.

* To serve, divide among 4 individual plates.

Nutritional Analysis per Serving

Calories 343 (Kilojoules 1,442); Total fat 5g; Saturated fat 1g; Protein 14g;
Cholesterol 3mg; Carbohydrates 60g; Sodium 182mg; Dietary fiber 6g;
Calories from fat 14%

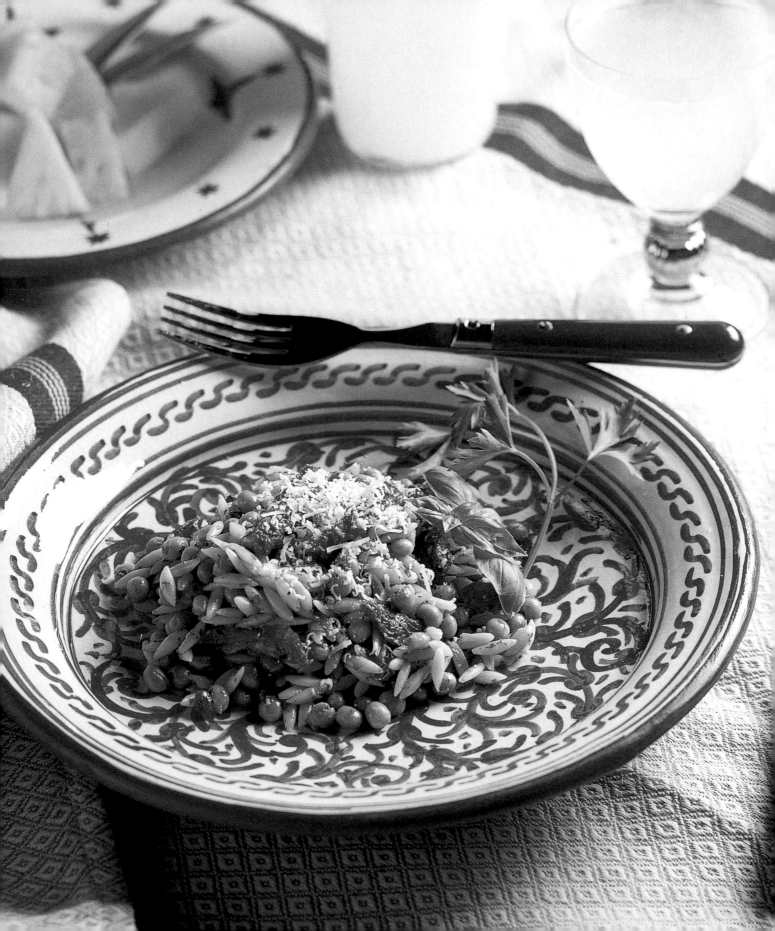

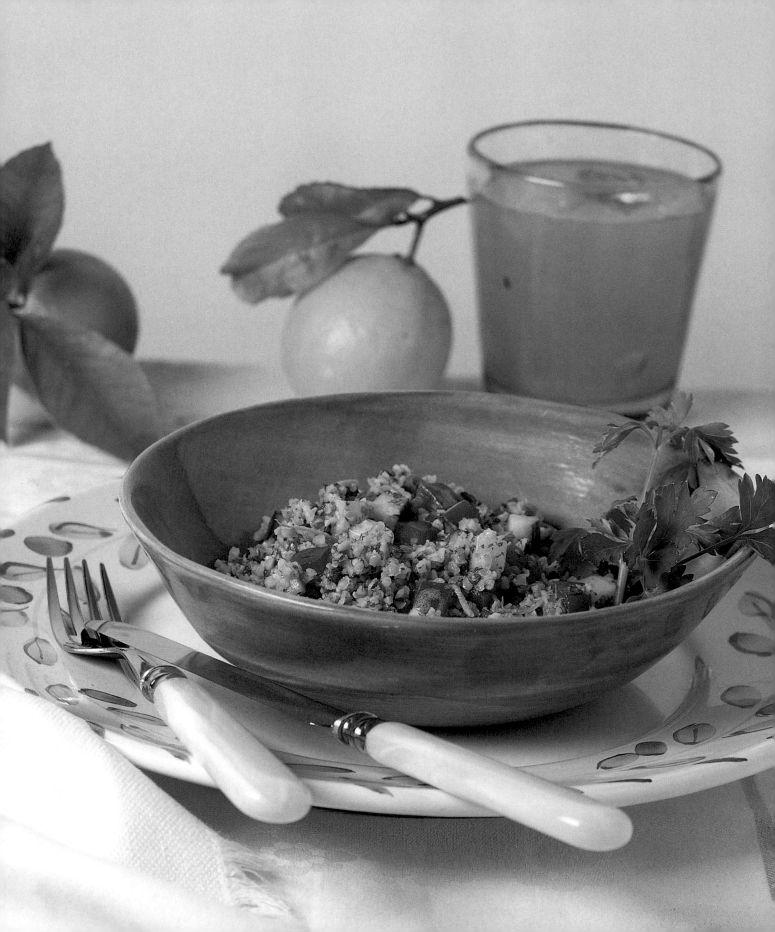

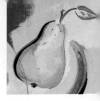

Tabbouleh

1 cup (6 oz/185 g) bulgur

1 tablespoon chopped fresh oregano

1 teaspoon ground cumin

¼ teaspoon salt

¼ teaspoon ground black pepper

1 cup (8 fl oz/250 ml) Chicken Stock
(recipe on page 206) or reduced
sodium chicken broth

1 cup (8 fl oz/250 ml) water

3 tablespoons lemon juice

3 tablespoons olive oil

2 tablespoons nonfat plain yogurt

2 garlic cloves, peeled and minced

4 green (spring) onions, green and
white parts, chopped

1 teaspoon finely grated lemon zest

1 cucumber (about 12 oz/375 g),
seeded and chopped

3 large tomatoes, seeded and chopped

¼ cup (⅓ oz/10 g) chopped
fresh flat-leaf (Italian) parsley

¼ cup (⅓ oz/10 g) chopped
fresh mint

fresh flat-leaf (Italian) parsley sprigs

Preparation: 20 minutes ✳ Cooking: 20 minutes ✳ Serves 4

At once robust, aromatic and refreshing, this salad is a classic of the Middle East. Bulgur, also known as cracked wheat, is flavorful and chewy and an excellent source of fiber. For variety, substitute other whole grains such as quinoa or barley.

✳ In a large bowl, combine the bulgur, oregano, cumin, salt and pepper and stir to mix well.

✳ In a small saucepan over medium-high heat, combine the stock or broth and the water and bring to a boil. Pour the boiling liquid over the bulgur mixture. Let stand until the liquid is absorbed, about 20 minutes.

✳ To make the dressing, in a small bowl, combine the lemon juice, olive oil, yogurt, garlic, green onions and lemon zest and whisk until blended.

✳ To the bulgur mixture, add the dressing, cucumber, tomatoes, chopped parsley and mint and toss to coat well.

✳ To serve, divide among 4 individual plates. Garnish with the parsley sprigs.

Nutritional Analysis per Serving

Calories 293 (Kilojoules 1,231); Total fat 11g; Saturated fat 2g; Protein 8g; Cholesterol 0mg; Carbohydrates 44g; Sodium 306mg; Dietary fiber 11g; Calories from fat 33%

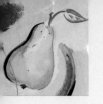

3 tablespoons crumbled goat cheese

2 tablespoons nonfat dairy sour cream

2 tablespoons nonfat milk

2 tablespoons chopped fresh chives

⅛ teaspoon ground black pepper

4 cups (8 oz/250 g) mixed salad
   greens

3 tomatoes (about 18 oz/560 g),
   seeded and sliced

1 red bell pepper (capsicum), roasted,
   peeled, seeded, deribbed and cut
   into strips

Cooking Tip

✳ To roast a pepper, whether a sweet bell
pepper or a hot pepper, cut the pepper
in half. Place on a baking sheet under a
broiler or hold over a gas flame, turning
often, until blackened, about 5 minutes.
Transfer to a paper bag, close and set aside
to cool, about 15 minutes. Using a small
knife, remove the skin, stem and seeds.

Greens and Peppers Salad

*Preparation: 15 minutes * Serves 4*

*Simple salad greens pack a lot of nutrition in fat-free, high-fiber form.
Chicory is rich in the B-vitamin folate and vitamins A and C, as well as
containing good amounts of calcium and potassium. Curly endive offers
folate and the antioxidant beta-carotene. Lamb's lettuce (mâche) is very
rich in vitamins A and C. More common lettuces contain varying but
significant amounts of folate and vitamins A and C, with Romaine (cos)
the richest source. Many well-stocked markets amd greengrocers today
sell mixed greens already trimmed, washed and bagged, ready to toss into
a salad bowl.*

✳ To make the dressing, in a small bowl, combine the goat
cheese, sour cream, milk, chives and pepper and whisk until
blended. The dressing can be stored in an airtight container for
up to 1 week.

✳ To serve, divide the greens among 4 individual plates. Top
each serving with an equal amount of the tomatoes, bell pepper
and dressing.

Nutritional Analysis per Serving

Calories 73 (Kilojoules 305); Total fat 3g; Saturated fat 1g; Protein 4g;
Cholesterol 5mg; Carbohydrates 10g; Sodium 59mg; Dietary fiber 3g;
Calories from fat 28%

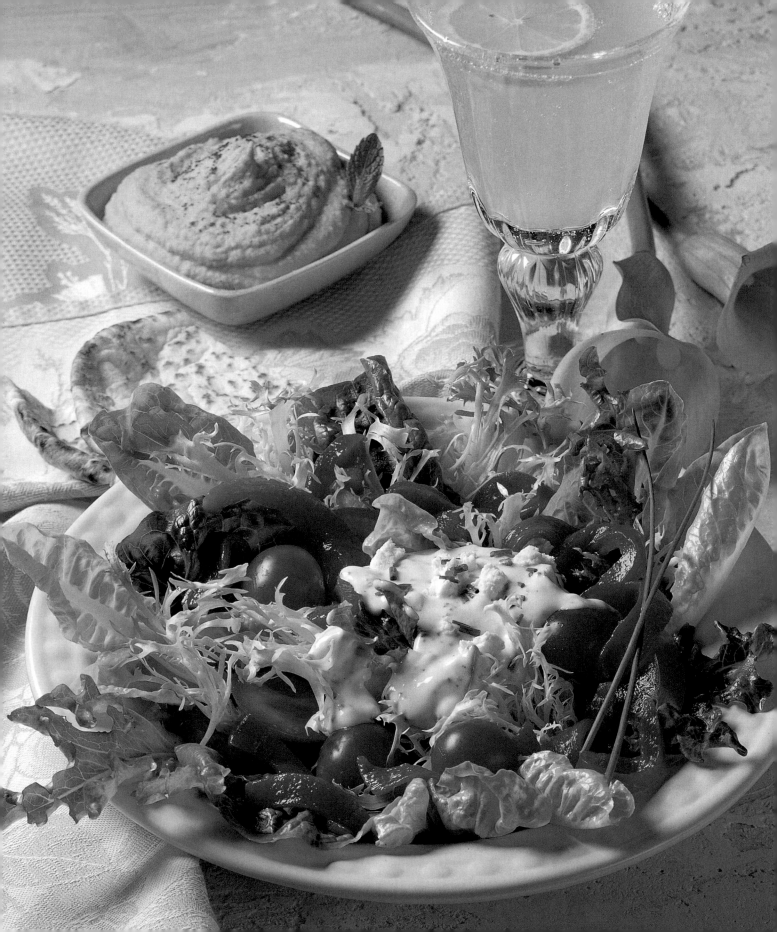

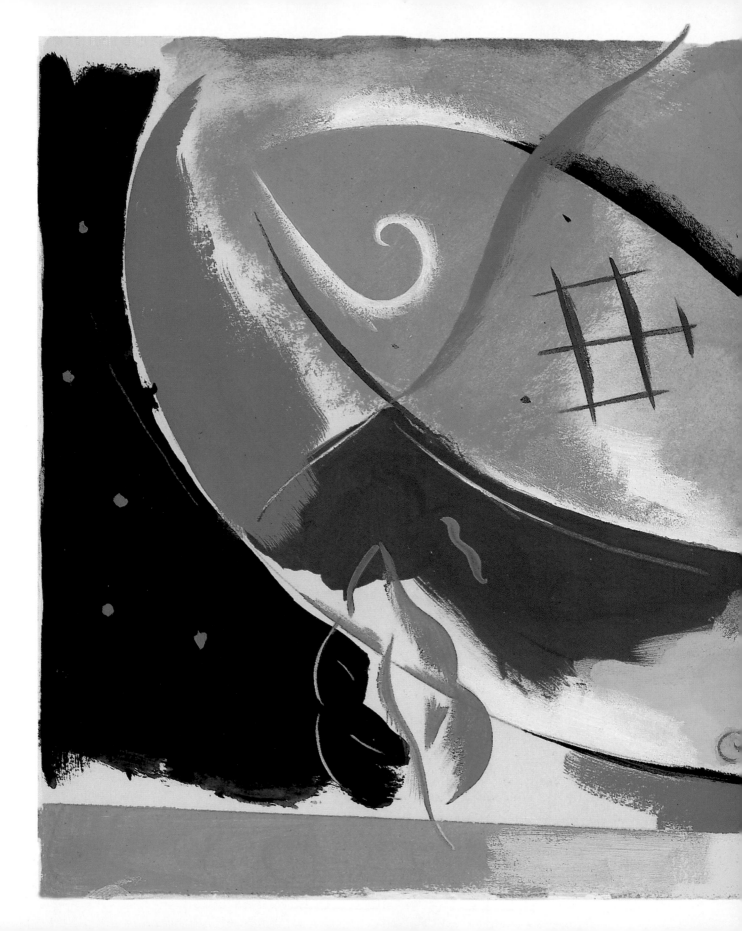

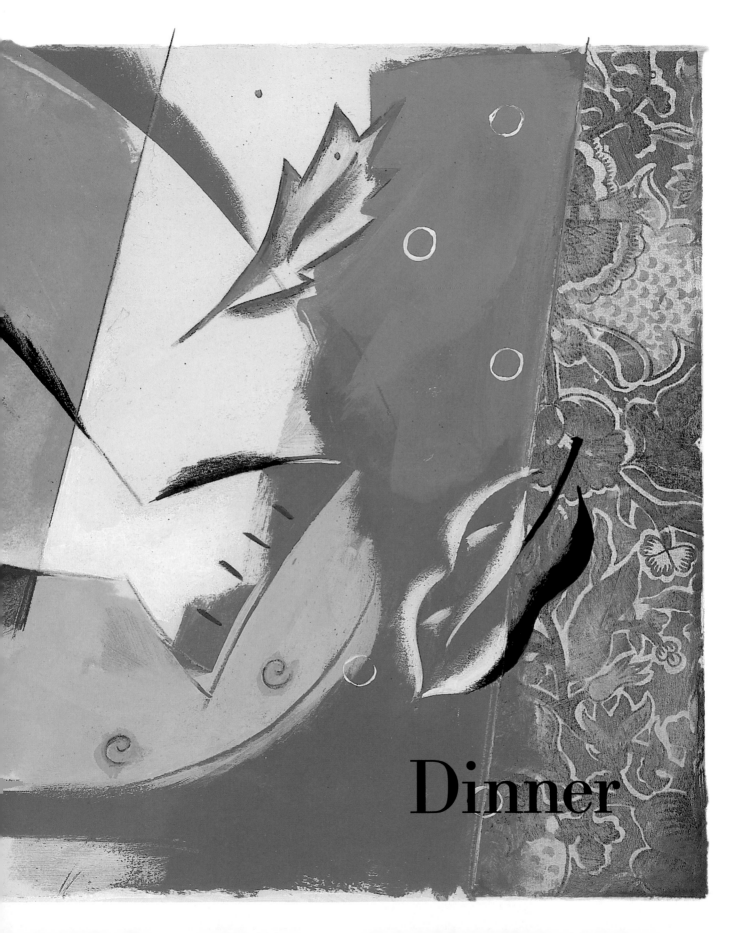

Dinner

Suggested Dinner Menus

Most of us are used to eating our biggest meal in the evening. However, the hours before we go to sleep are not necessarily the best time to eat large quantities of food. The menus shown here and the recipes on the following pages creatively address both these factors. They offer robust satisfaction through complex carbohydrates that fill us up while being low in fat, easy to digest and calming to the nervous system. The recipes also include protein in reduced portions and are so imaginatively seasoned, cooked and presented that a little goes a long way—one of the wisest strategies in any healthy eating regimen.

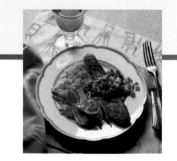

Salmon with Corn Sauce
page 132

Spring Vegetable Sauté
page 197

½ cup (2½ oz/75 g)
steamed brown rice

Summer Fruit in Rosemary Syrup
page 40

Nutritional Analysis per Serving: Calories 636 (Kilojoules 2,670); Total fat 12g; Saturated fat 2g; Protein 38g; Cholesterol 69mg; Carbohydrates 100g; Sodium 567mg; Dietary fiber 15g; Calories from fat 16%

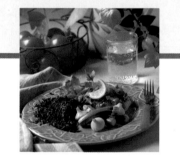

Red Snapper Puttanesca
page 135

½ cup (2½ oz/75 g) wild rice

½ cup (2½ oz/75 g)
steamed zucchini

Orange-Pecan Drop Cookies
page 216

Nutritional Analysis per Serving: Calories 516 (Kilojoules 2,165); Total fat 11g; Saturated fat 2g; Protein 36g; Cholesterol 58mg; Carbohydrates 71g; Sodium 617mg; Dietary fiber 6g; Calories from fat 19%

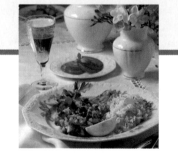

Trout with
Hazelnut-Shallot Sauce
page 136

Spicy Rice Pilaf
page 208

½ sliced tomato
with Mustard Vinaigrette
page 184

Cranberry-Applesauce
page 212

Nutritional Analysis per Serving: Calories 820 (Kilojoules 3,444); Total fat 21g; Saturated fat 3g; Protein 39g; Cholesterol 68mg; Carbohydrates 125g; Sodium 772mg; Dietary fiber 10g; Calories from fat 23%

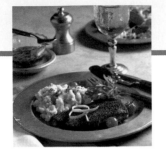

Blackened Catfish
page 139

Garlic Mashed Potatoes
page 205

1 cup (1 oz/30 g) mixed greens with ½ tomato and Sesame-Garlic Dressing
page 184

Apple-Walnut Bread
page 56

Nutritional Analysis per Serving: Calories 702 (Kilojoules 2,946); Total fat 21g; Saturated fat 4g; Protein 31g; Cholesterol 66mg; Carbohydrates 101g; Sodium 849mg; Dietary fiber 7g; Calories from fat 27%

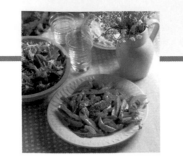

Sesame Chicken and Snow Peas in Apricot Sauce
page 140

½ cup (2 oz/60 g) angel hair pasta

1 cup (1 oz/30 g) mixed greens with Basil Dressing
page 183

Banana Cheesecake
page 235

Nutritional Analysis per Serving: Calories 675 (Kilojoules 2,834); Total fat 11g; Saturated fat 2g; Protein 43g; Cholesterol 98mg; Carbohydrates 103g; Sodium 654mg; Dietary fiber 6g; Calories from fat 14%

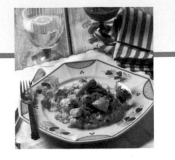

Curried Chicken Stew
page 143

½ cup (2½ oz/75 g) steamed brown rice

Lemon-Blueberry Ice Milk
page 224

Nutritional Analysis per Serving: Calories 419 (Kilojoules 1,760); Total fat 6g; Saturated fat 1g; Protein 34g; Cholesterol 69mg; Carbohydrates 58g; Sodium 314mg; Dietary fiber 6g; Calories from fat 13%

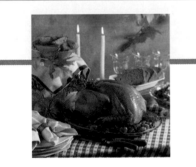

Roast Turkey
page 144

Bread and Apple Dressing
page 211

½ baked sweet potato

Spinach and Roasted Chestnuts
page 194

Pumpkin Spice Bread
page 231

Nutritional Analysis per Serving: Calories 1,189 (Kilojoules 4,994); Total fat 26g; Saturated fat 6g; Protein 71g; Cholesterol 184mg; Carbohydrates 168g; Sodium 1,286mg; Dietary fiber 13g; Calories from fat 20%

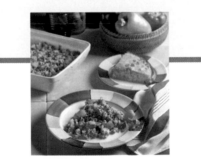

Mexican Chicken Casserole
page 147

Corn Pudding
page 201

Almond Gelatin Squares in Fruit
page 39

Nutritional Analysis per Serving: Calories 1,184 (Kilojoules 4,973); Total fat 20g; Saturated fat 4g; Protein 63g; Cholesterol 83mg; Carbohydrates 195g; Sodium 1,341mg; Dietary fiber 17g; Calories from fat 15%

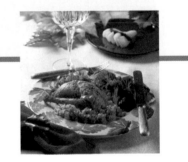

Roast Pheasant
page 148

Rice, Raisin and Rosemary Dressing
page 211

½ cup (1 oz/30 g) steamed broccoli

Pears with Chocolate Sauce
page 219

Nutritional Analysis per Serving: Calories 1,376 (Kilojoules 5,777); Total fat 29g; Saturated fat 8g; Protein 135g; Cholesterol 472mg; Carbohydrates 144g; Sodium 896mg; Dietary fiber 10g; Calories from fat 19%

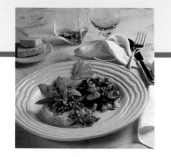

Garlic Pork Chops
with Black Mushrooms
page 151

*½ cup (2½ oz/75 g) steamed
snow peas*

Wild Rice with Mixed Dried Fruit
page 208

Almond Biscotti
page 215

Nutritional Analysis per Serving: Calories 623 (Kilojoules 2,616); Total fat 13g; Saturated fat 3g; Protein 39g; Cholesterol 95mg; Carbohydrates 86g; Sodium 983mg; Dietary fiber 7g; Calories from fat 19%

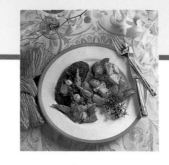

Filets Mignons with
Artichokes and Pearl Onions
page 152

Rosemary Roasted Potatoes
page 202

*1 celery stalk
with Chive-Chutney Dip*
page 186

Baked Apples
page 223

Nutritional Analysis per Serving: Calories 702 (Kilojoules 2,948); Total fat 21g; Saturated fat 5g; Protein 41g; Cholesterol 76mg; Carbohydrates 90g; Sodium 629mg; Dietary fiber 9g; Calories from fat 27%

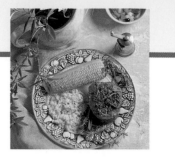

Bison Osso Buco
page 155

½ cup (2½ oz/75 g) steamed rice

1 corn on the cob

Melon and Blueberries in Sauce
page 220

Nutritional Analysis per Serving: Calories 693 (Kilojoules 2,910); Total fat 10g; Saturated fat 2g; Protein 59g; Cholesterol 140mg; Carbohydrates 91g; Sodium 1,098mg; Dietary fiber 5g; Calories from fat 13%

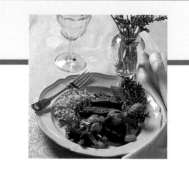

Grilled Bison
with Rosemary Marinade
page 156

Grilled Summer Vegetables
page 197

Orzo with Shallots and Herbs
page 205

Iced Cocoa
page 179

Nutritional Analysis per Serving: Calories 577 (Kilojoules 2,424); Total fat 8g; Saturated fat 2g; Protein 44g; Cholesterol 75mg; Carbohydrates 82g; Sodium 799mg; Dietary fiber 4g; Calories from fat 12%

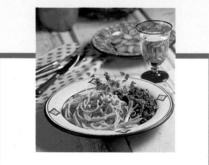

Spaghetti in Spicy Peanut Sauce
page 159

*½ cup (3½ oz/110 g)
steamed spinach*

*1 sliced cucumber with
Mustard Vinaigrette*
page 184

Banana Bread
page 52

Nutritional Analysis per Serving: Calories 758 (Kilojoules 3,184); Total fat 8g; Saturated fat 1g; Protein 24g; Cholesterol 0mg; Carbohydrates 149g; Sodium 709mg; Dietary fiber 10g; Calories from fat 10%

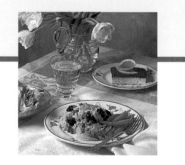

Lemon-Broccoli Risotto
page 160

Steamed Carrots with Dill
page 194

*1 cup (1 oz/30 g) mixed greens
with Sesame-Garlic Dressing*
page 184

Sponge Cake with
Chocolate-Orange Frosting
page 227

Nutritional Analysis per Serving: Calories 627 (Kilojoules 2,635); Total fat 14g; Saturated fat 2g; Protein 16g; Cholesterol 51mg; Carbohydrates 112g; Sodium 621mg; Dietary fiber 8g; Calories from fat 20%

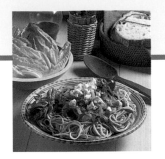

*Linguine with Goat Cheese,
Tomatoes and Onions*
page 163

*2 cups romaine lettuce
with Sesame-Garlic Dressing*
page 184

*Italian bread with
1 teaspoon margarine*

Raspberry Sherbet
page 224

Nutritional Analysis per Serving: Calories 760
(Kilojoules 3,191); Total fat 17g; Saturated fat 7g;
Protein 26g; Cholesterol 26mg; Carbohydrates 130g;
Sodium 517mg; Dietary fiber 13g; Calories from fat 20%

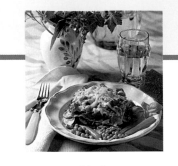

Vegetable Lasagna
page 164

*¼ cup (1 oz/30 g) each steamed
peas and carrots*

1 hard roll

Honey-Mint Fruit Compote
page 231

Nutritional Analysis per Serving: Calories 792
(Kilojoules 3,325); Total fat 11g; Saturated fat 4g;
Protein 42g; Cholesterol 24mg; Carbohydrates 132g;
Sodium 698mg; Dietary fiber 12g; Calories from fat 13%

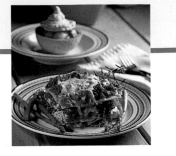

Bison Lasagna
page 167

5 spears steamed asparagus

2 bread sticks

Meringue-Topped Cantaloupe
page 228

Nutritional Analysis per Serving: Calories 845
(Kilojoules 3,549); Total fat 10g; Saturated fat 4g;
Protein 51g; Cholesterol 42mg; Carbohydrates 140g;
Sodium 526mg; Dietary fiber 14g; Calories from fat 11%

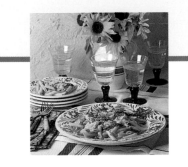

Penne with Garlic-Tomato Sauce
page 168

*1 slice French bread
with 1 teaspoon margarine*

*Poached Fruit with
Cinnamon-Yogurt Topping*
page 36

Nutritional Analysis per Serving: Calories 655
(Kilojoules 2,752); Total fat 10g; Saturated fat 1g;
Protein 21g; Cholesterol 4mg; Carbohydrates 122g;
Sodium 588mg; Dietary fiber 8g; Calories from fat 13%

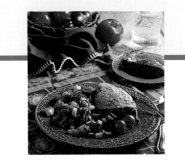

Spinach Soufflé
page 171

Ratatouille
page 198

Chocolate Cheesecake
page 236

Nutritional Analysis per Serving: Calories 684
(Kilojoules 2,871); Total fat 23g; Saturated fat 4g;
Protein 39g; Cholesterol 42mg; Carbohydrates 82g;
Sodium 913mg; Dietary fiber 8g; Calories from fat 30%

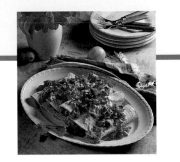

*Black Bean Enchiladas
with Tomato Salsa*
page 172

½ cup (2½ oz/75 g) steamed rice

2 carrots with Avocado Dressing
page 115

*Orange Custard
with Raspberry Sauce*
page 232

Nutritional Analysis per Serving: Calories 987
(Kilojoules 4,147); Total fat 22g; Saturated fat 6g;
Protein 38g; Cholesterol 224mg; Carbohydrates 166g;
Sodium 723mg; Dietary fiber 23g; Calories from fat 20%

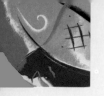

2 tablespoons reduced sodium
  soy sauce

2 garlic cloves, peeled and minced

1 tablespoon lemon juice

1 teaspoon sugar

4 center-cut salmon fillets, about
  4 oz (125 g) each

2 cups (12 oz/375 g) corn kernels

⅓ cup (2½ oz/75 g) chopped sun-
  dried tomatoes, packed without oil

½ cup (4 fl oz/125 ml) water

½ teaspoon ground cumin

¼ cup (¾ oz/20 g) chopped green
  (spring) onions, green and
  white parts

¼ cup (⅓ oz/10 g) chopped fresh
  cilantro (fresh coriander)

1 teaspoon ground black pepper

Storage Tip

✳ The Corn Sauce, which is also good
on chicken breasts or halibut, can be
made ahead, refrigerated in an airtight
container for up to 2 days and reheated
in a small saucepan over low heat while
the fish cooks.

Salmon with Corn Sauce

Preparation: 40 minutes ✳ Cooking: 20 minutes ✳ Serves 4

*When weather permits, cook the salmon on an outdoor charcoal grill for
a great summer dinner party. Although relatively high in fat as seafood
goes, salmon is a good source of omega-3 fatty acids, which benefit the
heart and circulatory system.*

✳ To make the marinade, in a shallow glass baking dish, combine
the soy sauce, garlic, lemon juice and sugar. Add the salmon
fillets, turn to coat both sides, cover, refrigerate and marinate
for 15 minutes to 8 hours.

✳ To make the sauce, in a small saucepan over medium-high
heat, combine the corn, tomatoes, water and cumin. Bring to a
boil, reduce the heat to low and simmer until the tomatoes are
soft, about 10 minutes. Remove from the heat, add the green
onions and cilantro and stir to mix well.

✳ In a large nonstick frying pan over medium-high heat, heat
1 tablespoon of the marinade. Transfer the salmon to a work
surface and coat with the pepper. Discard the remaining marinade.

✳ Add the salmon to the hot pan and sauté for 4 minutes. Turn
and sauté the fish until it just separates when pressed with a fork,
about 4 minutes more.

✳ To serve, divide the fillets among 4 individual plates. Top each
with an equal amount of the sauce.

Nutritional Analysis per Serving

Calories 317 (Kilojoules 1,331); Total fat 9g; Saturated fat 1g; Protein 32g;
Cholesterol 69mg; Carbohydrates 30g; Sodium 314mg; Dietary fiber 7g;
Calories from fat 25%

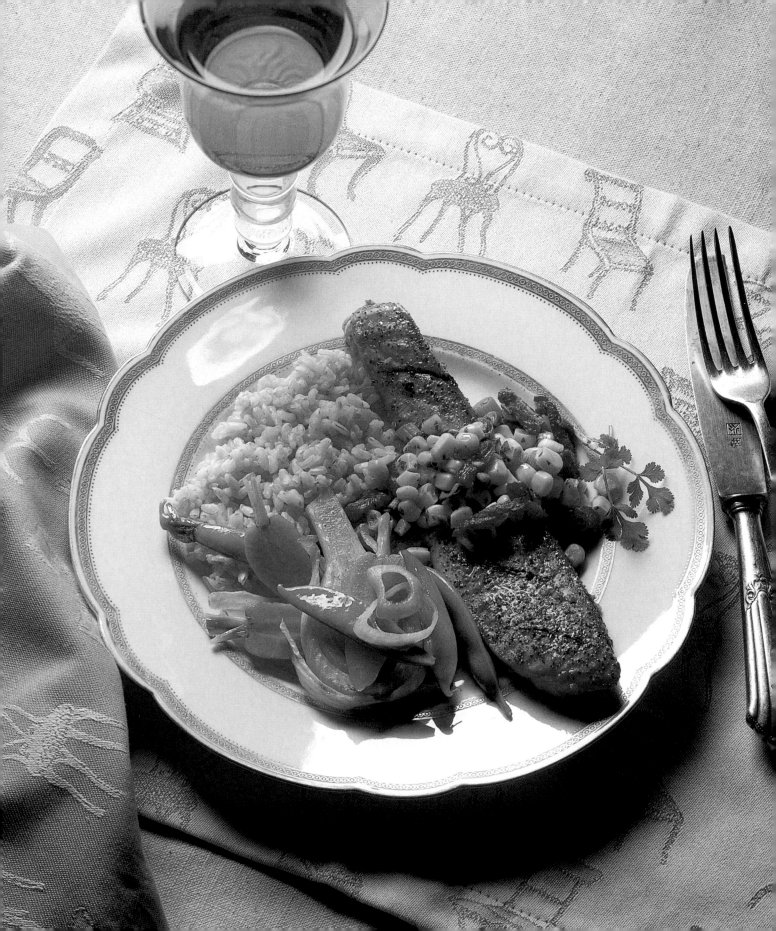

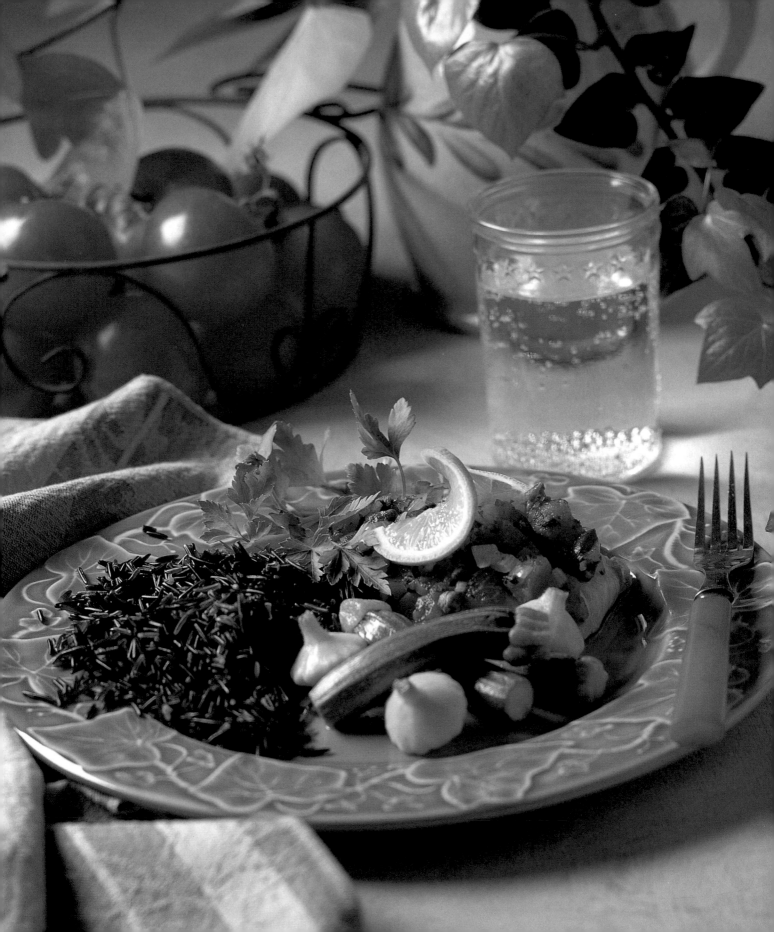

4 red snapper fillets, about 4 oz
   (125 g) each

1 tablespoon lemon juice

¼ teaspoon ground black pepper

2 teaspoons olive oil

1 onion, diced

3 garlic cloves, peeled and minced

3 large tomatoes, peeled and chopped

8 Niçoise olives, pitted and sliced

2 tablespoons drained capers

1 tablespoon minced anchovies

¼ cup (⅓ oz/10 g) chopped fresh basil

1 tablespoon chopped fresh oregano

1 bay leaf

¼ cup (⅓ oz/10 g) chopped fresh
   flat-leaf (Italian) parsley

½ lemon, cut into 4 wedges

4 fresh flat-leaf (Italian) parsley sprigs

Nutrition Tip

✳ Although garlic does not provide any significant quantities of nutrients, some medical studies have found that it contains certain substances that can reduce elevated blood cholesterol levels.

Red Snapper Puttanesca

Preparation: 25 minutes ✳ *Cooking: 40 minutes* ✳ *Serves 4*

Puttanesca is a traditional Italian sauce made with capers, olives, anchovies and tomatoes. The zesty combination of flavors pairs perfectly with the delicate taste and texture of red snapper. The sauce can also be spooned over grilled chicken or pasta for a light, healthy meal in minutes. Make the sauce ahead and refrigerate in an airtight container for up to 3 days.

✳ Preheat an oven to 350°F (180°C).

✳ Place the snapper fillets in a shallow glass baking dish and top with the lemon juice and pepper.

✳ To make the sauce, in a large nonstick frying pan over medium heat, heat the oil. Add the onion and garlic and sauté, stirring frequently, for 2 minutes. Add the tomatoes, olives, capers, anchovies, basil, oregano and bay leaf. Bring to a boil, reduce the heat to low and simmer for 5 minutes.

✳ Pour the sauce over the fillets and top with the chopped parsley. Cover with aluminum foil and bake until the fish just separates when pressed with a fork, about 30 minutes. Remove and discard the bay leaf.

✳ To serve, divide among 4 individual plates. Top each with a lemon wedge and a parsley sprig.

Nutritional Analysis per Serving

Calories 204 (Kilojoules 857); Total fat 6g; Saturated fat 1g; Protein 27g; Cholesterol 44mg; Carbohydrates 13g; Sodium 429mg; Dietary fiber 3g; Calories from fat 24%

½ cup (2½ oz/75 g) stone-ground
  yellow cornmeal (maize flour)
½ cup (2½ oz/75 g) whole wheat
  (wholemeal) bread crumbs
¼ cup (⅓ oz/10 g) chopped fresh
  flat-leaf (Italian) parsley
1 tablespoon finely grated lemon zest
½ teaspoon ground black pepper
3 garlic cloves, peeled and minced
1 cup (8 fl oz/250 ml) lowfat
  buttermilk
4 rainbow or brook trout fillets,
  about 4 oz (125 g) each
1 tablespoon hazelnut (filbert) oil
2 small shallots, peeled and chopped
¼ cup chopped hazelnuts (filberts)
¼ cup (2 fl oz/60 ml) Vegetable
  Stock (recipe on page 207) or
  vegetable broth
2 tablespoons lemon juice
½ lemon, cut into 4 wedges
4 fresh flat-leaf (Italian) parsley sprigs

Nutrition Tip

✳ Serve with lowfat accompaniments
(menu on page 128) to get a meal with
calories from fat below 25 percent.

Trout with Hazelnut-Shallot Sauce

Preparation: 20 minutes ✳ *Cooking: 30 minutes* ✳ *Serves 4*

Trout, like salmon, is rich in beneficial omega-3 fatty acids. The cornmeal coating and hazelnut sauce provide good fiber as well as adding distinctive flavor and crunchy texture. The breading is equally good on skinless chicken and turkey breast.

✳ Preheat an oven to 400°F (200°C). Coat a shallow glass baking dish with nonstick cooking spray.

✳ In a large shallow dish, combine the cornmeal, bread crumbs, chopped parsley, lemon zest, pepper and half of the garlic.

✳ Pour the buttermilk into another shallow dish. Add the trout and turn to coat both sides. Remove the fish from the buttermilk and place in the cornmeal mixture. Turn to coat both sides, pressing the mixture into the fish.

✳ Place the fish in the prepared dish and bake, uncovered, until it just separates when pressed with a fork, about 20 minutes.

✳ To make the sauce, in a medium nonstick frying pan over medium heat, heat the oil. Add the shallots and the remaining garlic and sauté for 2 minutes. Add the hazelnuts and sauté for 2 minutes more. Add the stock or broth and lemon juice and simmer for 5 minutes.

✳ To serve, divide among 4 individual plates. Top each with an equal amount of the sauce, a lemon wedge and a parsley sprig.

Nutritional Analysis per Serving

Calories 364 (Kilojoules 1,530); Total fat 14g; Saturated fat 2g; Protein 30g; Cholesterol 68mg; Carbohydrates 31g; Sodium 221mg; Dietary fiber 3g; Calories from fat 34%

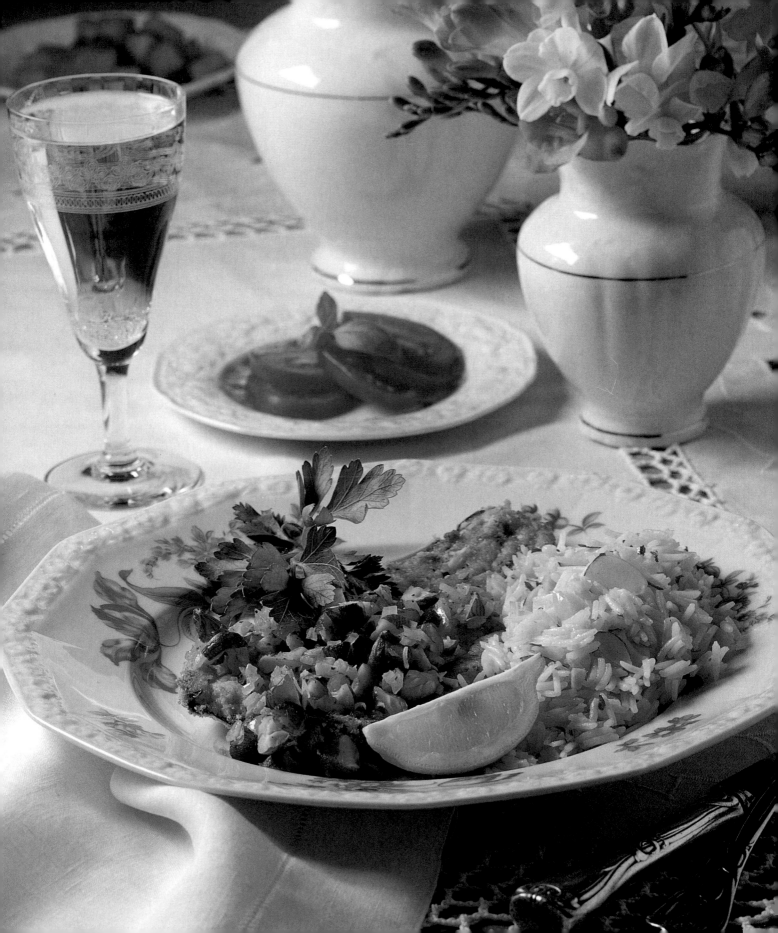

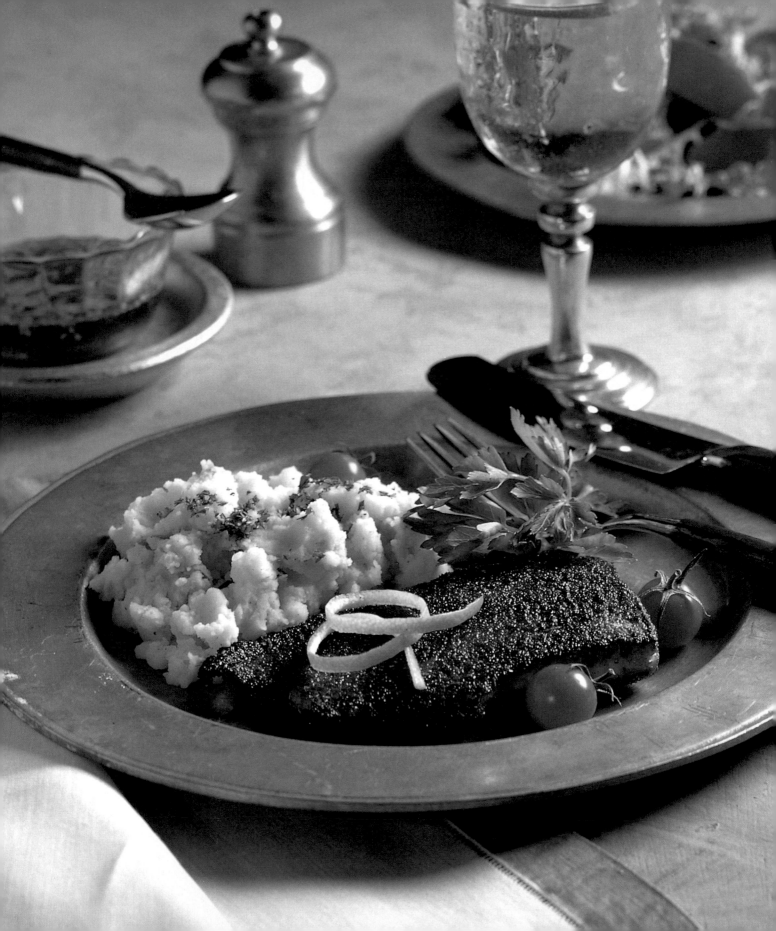

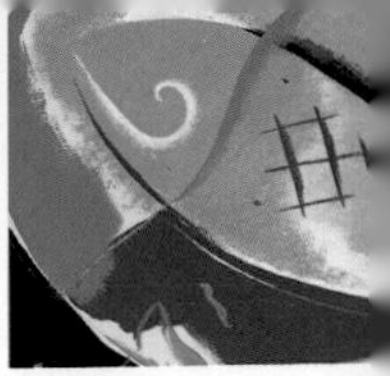

Blackened Catfish

2 teaspoons paprika
1 teaspoon cayenne pepper
1 teaspoon garlic powder
1 teaspoon dried thyme
½ teaspoon salt
1 teaspoon finely grated lemon zest
1 tablespoon olive oil
4 catfish fillets, about 4 oz (125 g) each
2 tablespoons lemon juice

Preparation: 10 minutes ✱ Cooking: 10 minutes ✱ Serves 4

The Cajun-style blackening technique is a terrific way to prepare these freshwater fish, and the same method can be used on other varieties of fish, skinless chicken breasts or pork chops. The spices blacken and season the fish as it cooks. Catfish is one of my favorite kinds of fish. Not only does it taste great, but it is an inexpensive source of protein.

✱ In a large shallow dish, combine the paprika, cayenne, garlic powder, thyme, salt and lemon zest. Add the catfish fillets and turn to coat both sides, pressing the herb-and-spice rub into the fish.

✱ In a large nonstick frying pan over medium-high heat, heat the oil.

✱ Add the fish and cook for 4 minutes. Pour the lemon juice over the fillets, turn and cook until the fish just separates when pressed with a fork, about 4 minutes more.

✱ To serve, divide among 4 individual plates.

Nutritional Analysis per Serving

Calories 185 (Kilojoules 777); Total fat 12g; Saturated fat 2g; Protein 17g; Cholesterol 37mg; Carbohydrates 2g; Sodium 313mg; Dietary fiber 0g; Calories from fat 57%

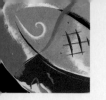

2 teaspoons dark sesame oil

3 garlic cloves, peeled and minced

1 lb (500 g) skinless, boneless chicken
   breast, cut into thin strips

1 tablespoon sesame seeds

⅓ cup (2 oz/60 g) sliced dried apricots

½ cup (4 fl oz/125 ml) water

½ cup (5 oz/155 g) apricot preserves

1 tablespoon reduced sodium soy sauce

1 tablespoon Dijon-style mustard

½ teaspoon grated fresh ginger

½ lb (250 g) snow peas (mangetouts),
   ends trimmed

Sesame Chicken and Snow Peas in Apricot Sauce

Preparation: 25 minutes ✳ *Cooking: 20 minutes* ✳ *Serves 4*

Apricots are an excellent source of beta-carotene, one of the antioxidants I encourage you to consume regularly for overall good health. Keep dried apricots on hand for snacks, especially in winter when the fresh ones are out of season. This sauce is so delicious that you'll want to try it without the chicken spooned over steamed vegetables or rice.

✳ In a large nonstick frying pan over medium heat, heat the oil. Add the garlic and sauté for 1 minute. Add chicken and sauté until browned and no longer pink in the center, about 5 minutes.

✳ Add the sesame seeds and sauté, stirring frequently, until browned, about 2 minutes. Add the apricots, water, apricot preserves, soy sauce, mustard and ginger and bring to a boil. Reduce the heat to low and simmer for 5 minutes. Add the snow peas and simmer until tender-crisp, about 5 minutes more.

✳ To serve, divide among 4 individual plates.

Nutritional Analysis per Serving

Calories 311 (Kilojoules 1,305); Total fat 5g; Saturated fat 1g; Protein 29g; Cholesterol 66mg; Carbohydrates 38g; Sodium 332mg; Dietary fiber 3g; Calories from fat 14%

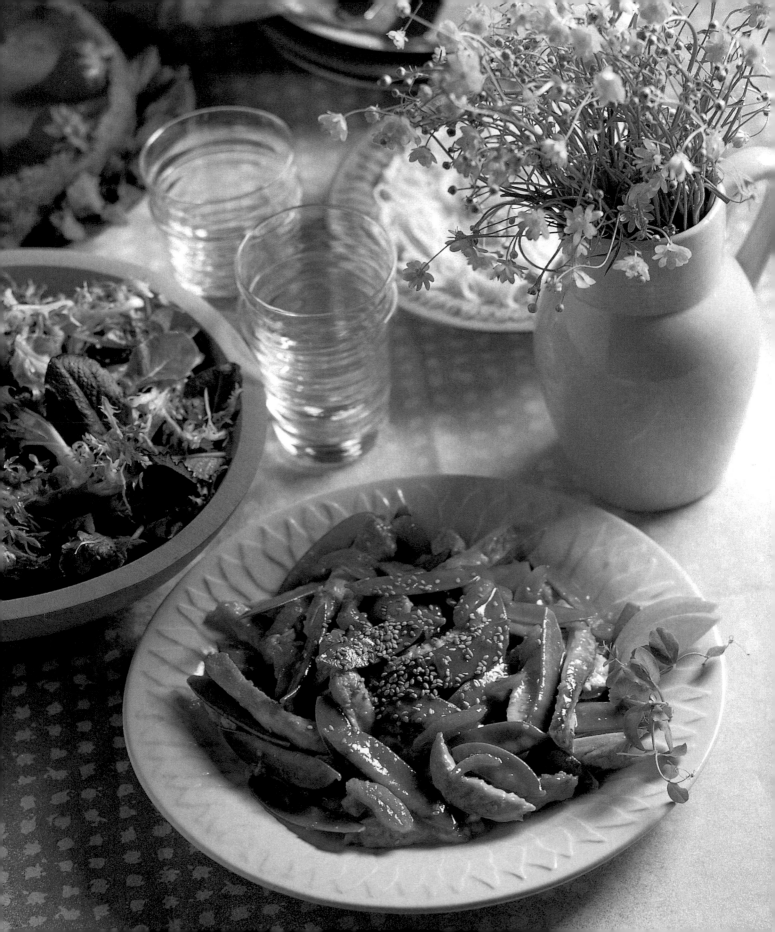

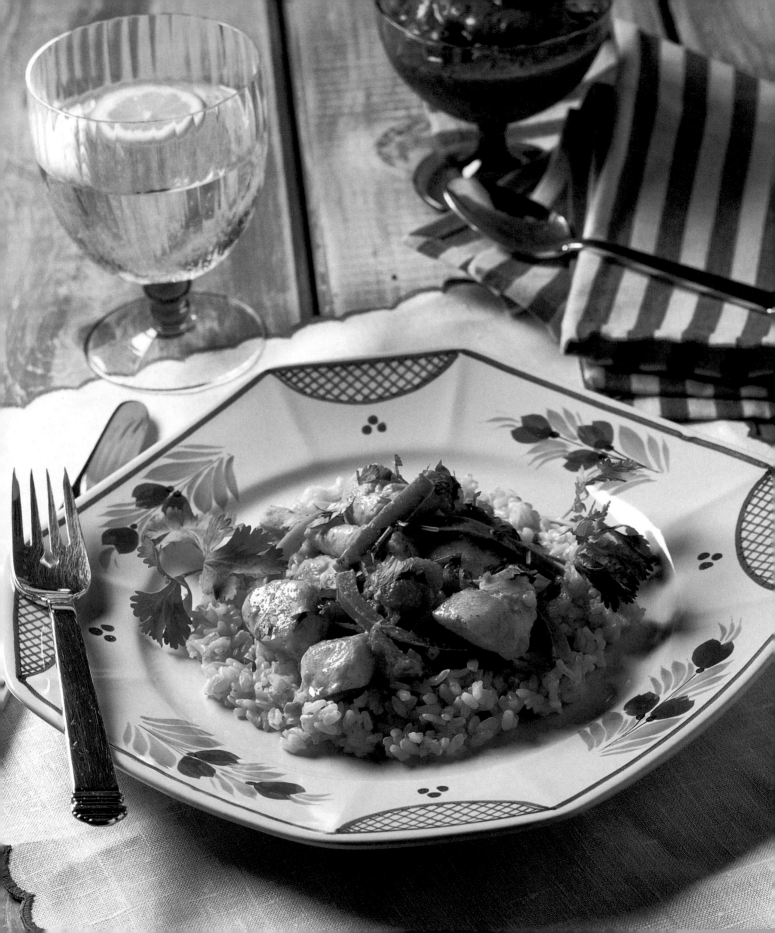

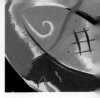

2 teaspoons olive oil

1 onion, chopped

3 garlic cloves, peeled and minced

1 green bell pepper (capsicum), seeded, deribbed and sliced into thin strips

1 lb (500 g) boneless, skinless chicken breast, cut into 1-inch (2.5-cm) pieces

4 large tomatoes, peeled, seeded and chopped

1½ teaspoons curry powder

1 teaspoon ground cumin

1 teaspoon ground turmeric

¼ teaspoon ground ginger

¼ teaspoon salt

¼ teaspoon ground black pepper

⅓ cup (2½ oz/75 g) nonfat plain yogurt

2 tablespoons chopped fresh cilantro (fresh coriander)

Shopping Tip

✳ Fresh cilantro, sometimes called Chinese parsley, adds a unique piquancy to this Asian-spiced stew. If fresh cilantro is not available, use flat-leaf (Italian) parsley instead. For the best spices, seek out a source such as an ethnic market or the mail-order firm listed in the Resources Guide on page 240.

Curried Chicken Stew

Preparation: 30 minutes ✳ Cooking: 25 minutes ✳ Serves 4

The mild, intriguing curry sauce also works well with chunks of lean pork tenderloin, cooked in the same way.

✳ In a large nonstick frying pan over medium heat, heat the oil. Add the onion, garlic and bell pepper and sauté for 2 minutes. Add the chicken and sauté until browned and no longer pink in the center, about 5 minutes. Add the tomatoes, curry, cumin, turmeric, ginger, salt and pepper. Bring to a boil, reduce the heat to low and simmer for 15 minutes. Remove from the heat and add the yogurt and cilantro. Stir to mix well.

✳ To serve, divide among 4 individual plates.

Nutritional Analysis per Serving

Calories 218 (Kilojoules 915); Total fat 5g; Saturated fat 0g; Protein 30g; Cholesterol 66mg; Carbohydrates 15g; Sodium 239mg; Dietary fiber 3g; Calories from fat 19%

Roast Turkey

1 turkey, about 10 lb (5 kg)

½ tablespoon salt

½ tablespoon ground black pepper

2 tablespoons margarine, melted

2 tablespoons chopped fresh rosemary

2 tablespoons chopped fresh thyme

2 tart apples, such as Granny Smith or pippin, cored and sliced

1 onion, sliced

Storage Tip

✳ To store fresh herbs, trim their stems slightly; place in a jar or other container of fresh water, as you would cut flowers; and refrigerate. Trim the stems and freshen the water daily. The herbs should keep for up to 1 week.

Preparation: 15 minutes ✳ *Cooking: 3 hours 20 minutes* ✳ *Serves 6*

To ensure proper cooking of a turkey, plan on about 20 minutes per pound for an unstuffed bird. I never cook stuffing or dressing inside poultry as it will absorb fat. If you're using an instant-read thermometer, do not insert it into the meat while it roasts; just use to test for doneness.

✳ Preheat an oven to 450°F (230°C). Coat the rack of a large roasting pan with nonstick cooking spray. Remove the giblets, heart, liver and neck from inside the turkey and reserve for another use.

✳ Rinse the bird inside and out, pat dry and sprinkle inside and out with the salt and pepper. Place the turkey, breast side up, on the rack in the pan.

✳ In a small bowl, combine the margarine, rosemary and thyme. Brush the turkey with the herb mixture. Insert a meat thermometer deep into the thickest part of the thigh, next to the body but not touching the bone. Spread the apple and onion slices around the bird.

✳ Place the turkey in the oven and immediately reduce the temperature to 350°F (180°C). Roast, basting every 15 minutes with the pan drippings, until the thermometer registers 175°F (75°C) and a drumstick moves easily in the joint, about 3 hours and 20 minutes.

✳ Transfer to a platter and discard the onion and apples. Cover the turkey with foil and let rest for 10–15 minutes. Remove the skin, carve and serve. One serving is 6 oz (185 g).

Nutritional Analysis per Serving

Calories 286 (Kilojoules 1,200); Total fat 8g; Saturated fat 3g; Protein 50g; Cholesterol 131mg; Carbohydrates 0g; Sodium 126mg; Dietary fiber 0g; Calories from fat 26%

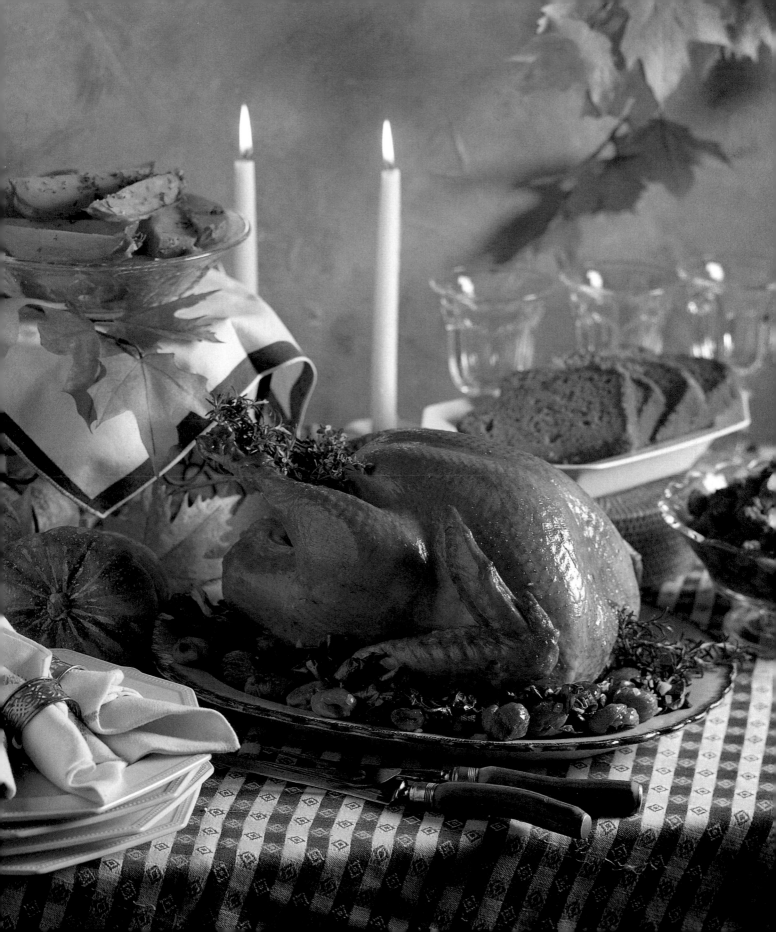

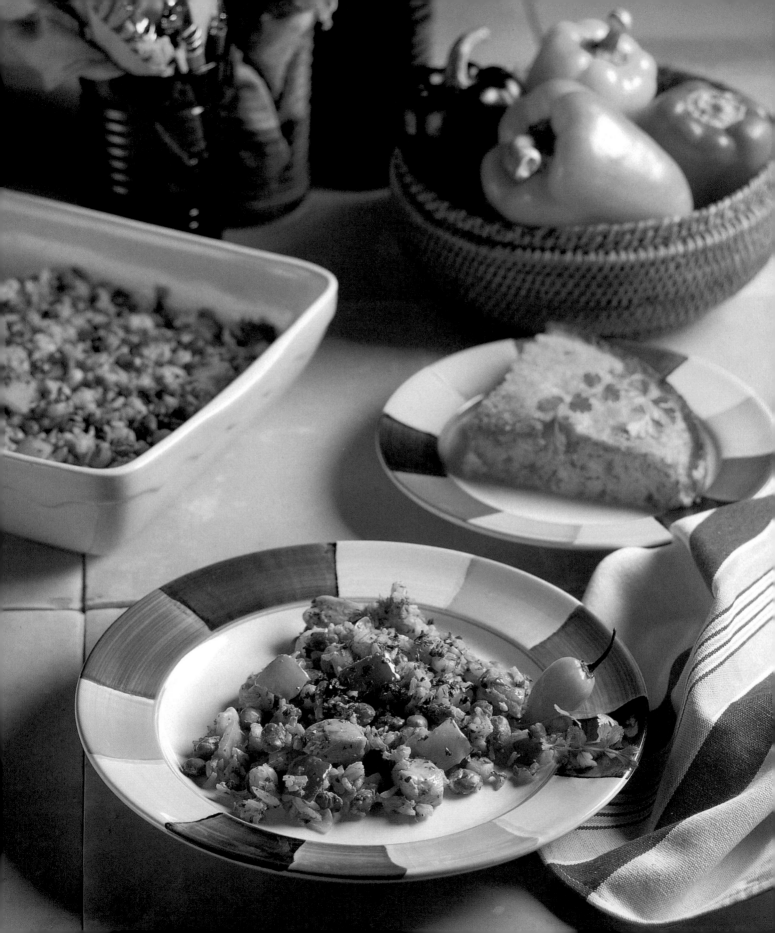

Mexican Chicken Casserole

*Preparation: 25 minutes * Cooking: 1 hour * Serves 4*

The combination of peppers, chili powder and pinto beans inspired the name of this easy-to-put-together dish, originally made from leftovers Karen Averitt had around the kitchen in Montana. I loved the taste and asked her to figure out what she had used so she could contribute it to this book. The casserole can be assembled ahead, covered with plastic wrap and refrigerated for up to 2 days before baking.

1 lb (500 g) boneless, skinless chicken breast, cut into 1-inch (2.5-cm) pieces

1 red bell pepper (capsicum), seeded, deribbed and chopped

1 yellow bell pepper (capsicum), seeded, deribbed and chopped

1 onion, chopped

4 garlic cloves, peeled and minced

1 tablespoon cumin seeds

1 tablespoon chopped fresh oregano

1 teaspoon chili powder

¼ teaspoon salt

¼ teaspoon ground black pepper

2 large tomatoes, peeled, seeded and chopped

14 oz (440 g) canned yellow hominy

1½ cups (7 oz/220 g) cooked pinto beans

1½ cups (7½ oz/235 g) cooked rice

¼ cup (⅓ oz/10 g) chopped fresh cilantro (fresh coriander)

¼ cup (2 oz/60 g) nonfat dairy sour cream

* Preheat an oven to 350°F (180°C). Coat a 13-by-9-by-2-inch (33-by-23-by-5-cm) baking dish with nonstick cooking spray.

* Coat a large nonstick frying pan with nonstick cooking spray and place over medium heat. Add the chicken, bell peppers, onion, garlic, cumin seeds, oregano, chili powder, salt and pepper and sauté, stirring frequently, until the chicken is golden, about 5 minutes. Add the tomatoes and simmer for 5 minutes. Add the hominy, pinto beans and rice and cook for 5 minutes more.

* Remove from the heat and add the cilantro and sour cream. Stir to mix well.

* Transfer to the prepared dish and bake until bubbly, about 45 minutes.

* To serve, divide among 4 individual plates.

Nutritional Analysis per Serving

Calories 400 (Kilojoules 1,682); Total fat 4g; Saturated fat 1g; Protein 36g; Cholesterol 66mg; Carbohydrates 55g; Sodium 448mg; Dietary fiber 7g; Calories from fat 9%

3 tablespoons chopped fresh sage

1 teaspoon paprika

1 teaspoon ground fennel seeds

¼ teaspoon cayenne pepper

¼ teaspoon ground black pepper

2 pheasants, about 3 lb (1.5 kg) each, rinsed and halved

1 tablespoon olive oil

1 small onion, chopped

3 garlic cloves, peeled and minced

1 cup (8 fl oz/250 ml) Chicken Stock (recipe on page 206) or reduced sodium chicken broth

2 shallots, peeled and minced

¼ cup (2 fl oz/60 ml) balsamic vinegar

2 tablespoons nonfat dairy sour cream

Roast Pheasant

Preparation: 30 minutes ✳ Cooking: 1 hour 20 minutes ✳ Serves 4

Game birds are lower in fat than chicken or turkey and contain none of the additives found in some brands of commercial poultry. We think the spices in this recipe really bring out the distinctive flavor of the pheasant. If pheasant isn't available, substitute game hens, capon or chicken.

✳ Preheat an oven to 350°F (180°C). Coat a shallow glass baking dish with nonstick cooking spray.

✳ In a small bowl, combine the sage, paprika, fennel, cayenne and pepper. Rub the mixture evenly over the pheasants.

✳ In a large nonstick frying pan over medium heat, heat the oil. Add the onion and half of the garlic and sauté, stirring frequently, until the onion is soft, about 2 minutes. Add pheasants and sauté for 5 minutes. Turn and sauté until browned, about 5 minutes more.

✳ Transfer the pheasants to the prepared dish and top with half of the stock or broth. Roast, uncovered, basting with the pan juices every 15 minutes, until the juices run clear when the meat is pierced with a knife, 35–45 minutes.

✳ To make the sauce, coat the inside of a small saucepan with nonstick cooking spray and place over medium heat. Add the shallots and the remaining garlic and sauté for 2 minutes. Add the balsamic vinegar and the remaining stock or broth, bring to a boil, reduce the heat to low and simmer until the sauce is reduced slightly and the shallots are soft, about 10 minutes.

✳ Transfer the pheasants to a serving platter and reserve the pan juices. Raise the heat under the sauce to medium. Add the pan juices and whisk until blended and simmering. Remove from the heat and whisk in the sour cream.

✳ To serve, remove the skin and top the meat with the sauce.

Nutritional Analysis per Serving

Calories 757 (Kilojoules 3,178); Total fat 23g; Saturated fat 7g; Protein 124g; Cholesterol 471mg; Carbohydrates 6g; Sodium 340mg; Dietary fiber 1g; Calories from fat 28%

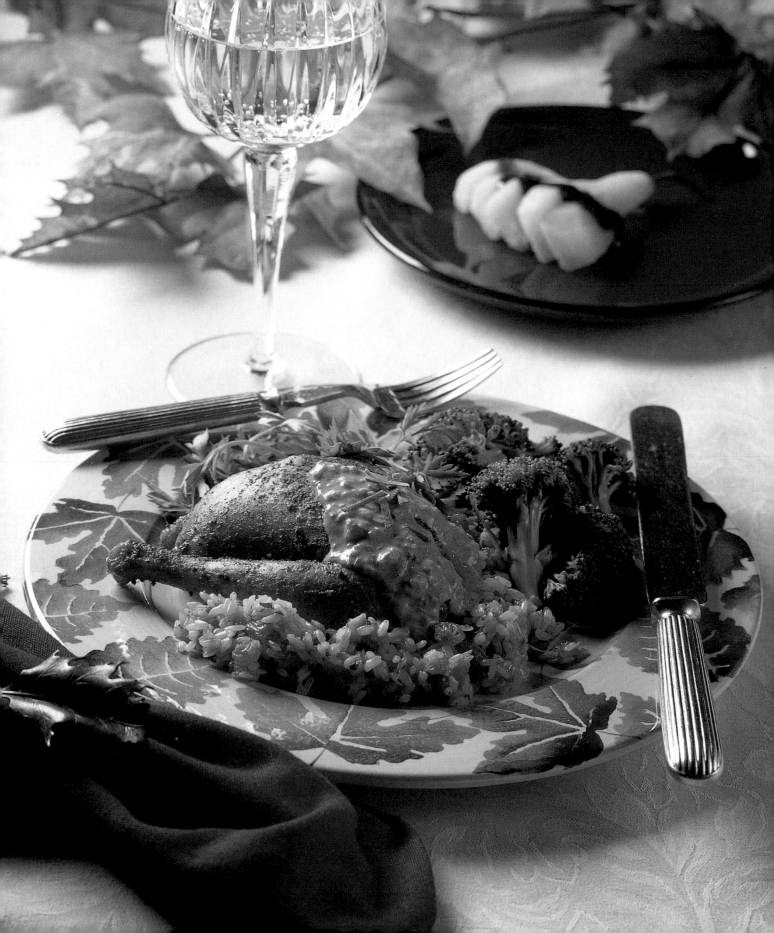

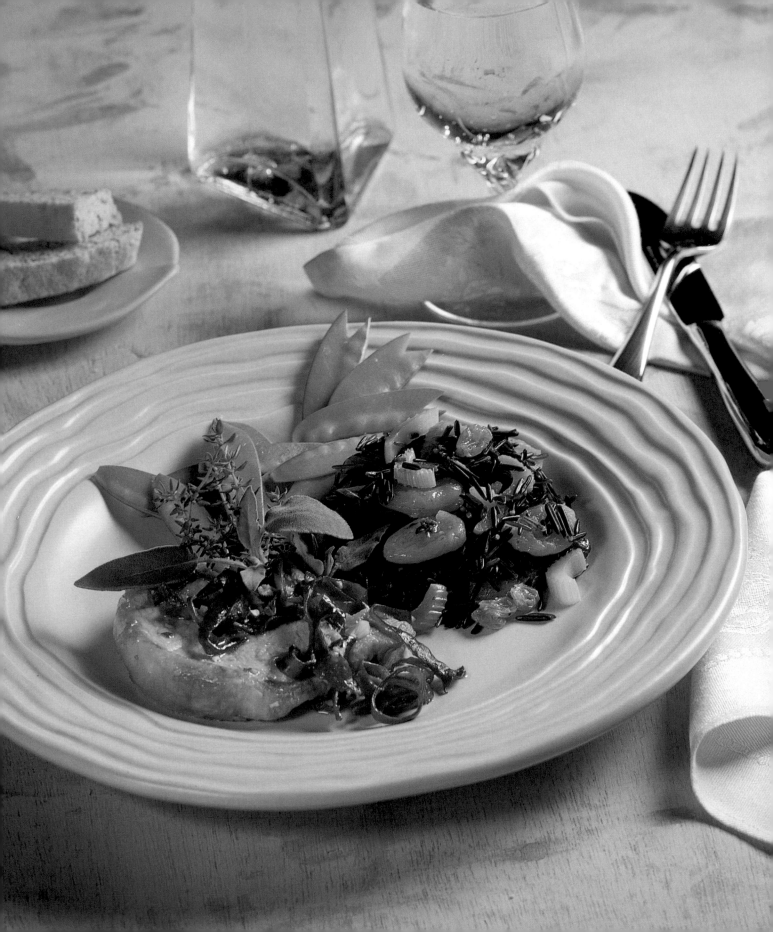

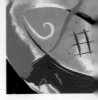

Garlic Pork Chops with Black Mushrooms

Preparation: 25 minutes ✳ Cooking: 30 minutes ✳ Serves 4

Black (cloud ear) mushrooms are usually sold dried and can be found in most supermarkets and specialty-food stores or in Asian markets. If you find neither those nor shiitake mushrooms, substitute fresh button mushrooms. The sauce will not be as richly flavored, but the overall dish will still be delicious.

1 cup (8 fl oz/250 ml) Chicken Stock (recipe on page 206) or reduced sodium chicken broth

1 oz (30 g) dried black (cloud ear) mushrooms or dried shiitake mushrooms, stemmed

¼ cup (2 fl oz/60 ml) rice wine vinegar

2 tablespoons reduced sodium soy sauce

2 tablespoons honey

¼ teaspoon hot pepper flakes

2 teaspoons dark sesame oil

4 garlic cloves, peeled and minced

1 tablespoon minced fresh ginger

4 boneless pork loin chops, about 4 oz (125 g) each, trimmed of visible fat

✳ In a small saucepan over medium heat, bring the stock or broth to a boil. Add the mushrooms, reduce the heat to low and simmer, uncovered, for 10 minutes.

✳ In a small bowl, combine the vinegar, soy sauce, honey and pepper flakes.

✳ In a large nonstick frying pan over medium heat, heat the sesame oil. Add the garlic and ginger and sauté, stirring frequently, for 2 minutes. Add the chops and cook for 2 minutes. Turn and cook until browned, about 2 minutes more. Add the vinegar mixture and bring to a boil. Reduce the heat to low and simmer for 5 minutes.

✳ Using a slotted spoon, remove the mushrooms from the stock or broth and slice into thin strips. Reserve the liquid.

✳ Stir the mushrooms and reserved liquid into the pan with the chops, reduce the heat to low and simmer until the sauce is reduced and the chops are no longer pink in the center, about 5 minutes.

✳ To serve, divide the chops among 4 individual plates. Top each with an equal amount of the mushroom sauce.

Nutrition Tip

✳ Purchase cuts with *loin* or *leg* in the name; these are the leanest. Today's selection of pork products fits perfectly into a healthy lifestyle. These lean cuts trimmed of visible fat are 31 percent lower in fat and 14 percent lower in calories compared with the pork of just a decade ago.

Nutritional Analysis per Serving

Calories 249 (Kilojoules 1,045); Total fat 8g; Saturated fat 2g; Protein 27g; Cholesterol 71mg; Carbohydrates 16g; Sodium 519mg; Dietary fiber 1g; Calories from fat 30%

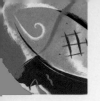

6 cups (48 fl oz/1.5 l) water

¾ lb (375 g) pearl onions

1 tablespoon olive oil

5 artichoke hearts, quartered

1 red bell pepper (capsicum), seeded,
    deribbed and thinly sliced

1 tablespoon chopped fresh thyme

½ tablespoon black peppercorns,
    cracked

4 filets mignons, about 4 oz (125 g)
    each, trimmed of visible fat

¼ cup (⅓ oz/10 g) chopped fresh
    flat-leaf (Italian) parsley

Nutrition Tip

✻ The recipe was designed using fresh or
frozen artichoke hearts. If only marinated
ones are available, drain and rinse them
before using to reduce the fat from the
oily marinade.

Filets Mignons with Artichokes and Pearl Onions

Preparation: 25 minutes ✻ Cooking: 20 minutes ✻ Serves 4

When shopping for filets mignons, choose cuts with little visible fat and a bright red color. Before cooking, trim any visible fat. A 4-oz (125-g) filet mignon will cook down to a 3-oz (90-g) serving, about the size of a deck of cards. Combine this main course with dishes that are very lowfat if you desire a meal with calories from fat of less than 25 percent.

✻ In a medium saucepan over high heat, bring the water to a boil. Add the onions and blanch for 5 minutes. Drain, rinse in cold water and remove the outer skin.

✻ In a large nonstick frying pan over medium heat, heat the olive oil. Add the onions, artichokes, bell pepper and thyme and sauté, stirring frequently, until the onions and artichokes are golden and the bell pepper is tender-crisp, about 10 minutes. Using a slotted spoon, remove the vegetables from the pan and keep warm.

✻ Press the cracked pepper into both sides of the filets mignons.

✻ Place the steaks in the hot pan and cook for 5 minutes. Turn and cook until the meat is dark brown on the outside and slightly pink in the center for medium-rare, 3–5 minutes more.

✻ To serve, divide the filets among 4 individual plates. Top each with an equal amount of the vegetable mixture and parsley.

Nutritional Analysis per Serving

Calories 266 (Kilojoules 1,117); Total fat 13g; Saturated fat 4g; Protein 26g;
Cholesterol 70mg; Carbohydrates 12g; Sodium 91mg; Dietary fiber 2g;
Calories from fat 43%

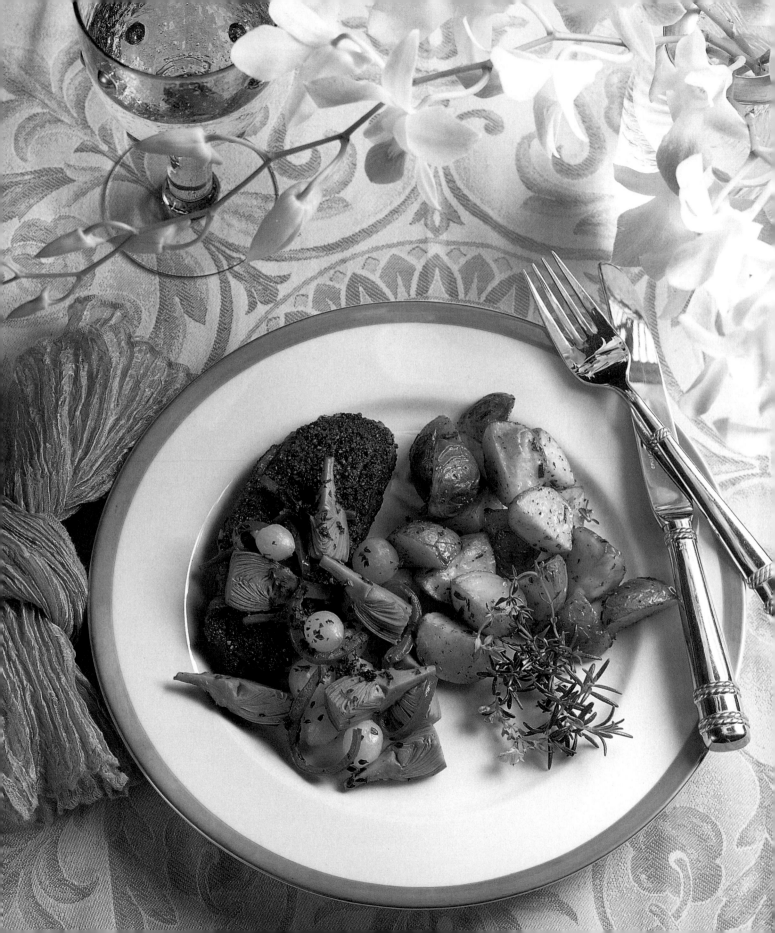

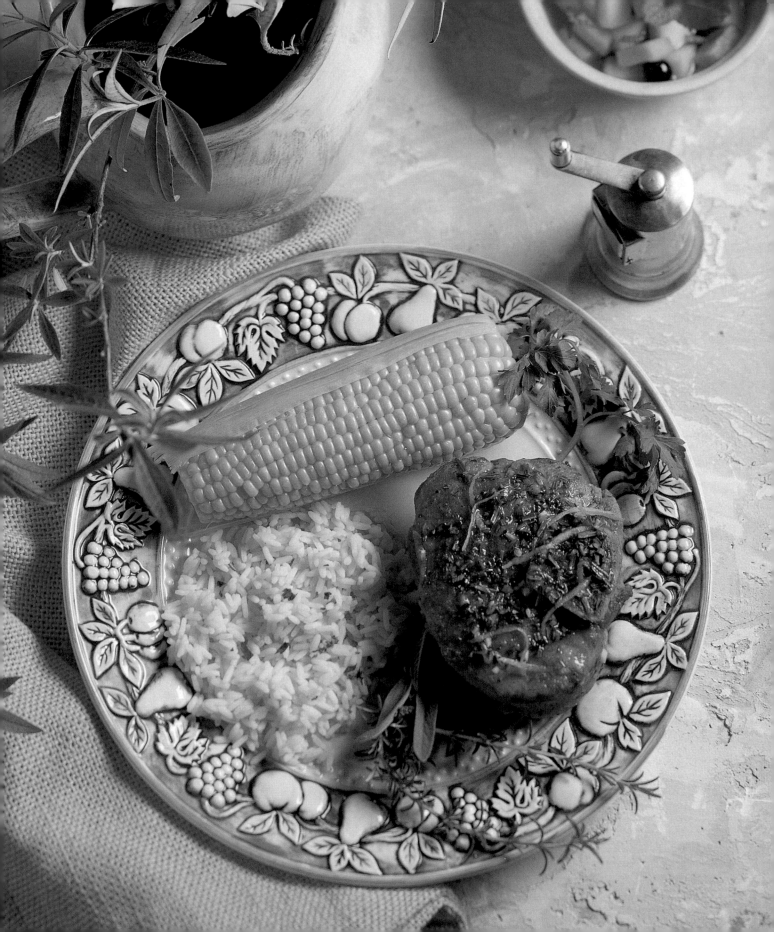

Bison Osso Buco

Preparation: 20 minutes ✳ *Cooking: 3 hours 10 minutes* ✳ *Serves 4*

This is actually our favorite special-occasion meal. Slow cooking on low heat makes this relatively inexpensive cut of meat quite tender. Check the Resources Guide on page 240 for mail-order sources of bison meat. You'll be amazed at the wonderful taste of such a lowfat meat. Substitute beef chuck or rump roast or veal, if desired, bearing in mind that their fat contents may be different than that shown for the bison.

½ cup (2½ oz/75 g) unbleached flour

1 teaspoon dried oregano

1 teaspoon dried basil

1 teaspoon dried rosemary

1 teaspoon dried sage

1 teaspoon salt

1 teaspoon ground black pepper

4 lb (2 kg) bison shanks or veal shanks, trimmed of visible fat and cut into 2-inch (5-cm) pieces

1 tablespoon olive oil

¼ cup (⅓ oz/10 g) chopped fresh rosemary

¼ cup (⅓ oz/10 g) chopped fresh sage

2 tablespoons finely grated lemon zest

8 garlic cloves, peeled and minced

½ cup (4 fl oz/125 ml) balsamic vinegar

3 cups (24 fl oz/750 ml) Chicken Stock (recipe on page 206) or reduced sodium chicken broth

¼ cup (⅓ oz/10 g) chopped fresh flat-leaf (Italian) parsley

✳ In a shallow glass baking dish, combine the flour, dried oregano, basil, rosemary, sage, salt and pepper. Add the bison or veal shanks and turn to coat well.

✳ In a 4-qt (4-l) Dutch oven over medium heat, heat the oil. Add the bison or veal and sauté, stirring frequently, until browned, about 5 minutes. Add the fresh rosemary and sage, lemon zest and garlic and sauté, stirring frequently, for 2 minutes more. Add the vinegar and 1 cup (8 fl oz/250 ml) of the stock or broth and simmer, uncovered, until the liquid is almost evaporated, about 20 minutes. Add the remaining stock or broth, cover, reduce the heat to low and simmer for 40 minutes more.

✳ Preheat an oven to 350°F (180°C).

✳ Cover the bison or veal and bake for 2 hours, spooning the sauce over the meat every 15 minutes.

✳ To serve, divide among 4 individual plates. Top each with an equal amount of the parsley.

Nutrition Tip

✳ The marrow from the center of the shank—a traditional delicacy enjoyed with osso buco—is very high in fat and should not be eaten as part of this recipe.

Nutritional Analysis per Serving

Calories 377 (Kilojoules 1,585); Total fat 8g; Saturated fat 2g; Protein 52g; Cholesterol 140mg; Carbohydrates 19g; Sodium 1,072mg; Dietary fiber 1g; Calories from fat 20%

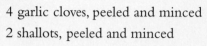

4 garlic cloves, peeled and minced

2 shallots, peeled and minced

¼ cup (⅓ oz/10 g) chopped fresh
flat-leaf (Italian) parsley

¼ cup (⅓ oz/10 g) chopped fresh
rosemary

½ cup (4 fl oz/125 ml) reduced
sodium beef broth

2 tablespoons reduced sodium
soy sauce

¼ cup (2 fl oz/60 ml) lemon juice

1 tablespoon finely grated lemon zest

½ tablespoon black peppercorns

1 lb (500 g) bison tenderloin or beef
sirloin, trimmed of visible fat

Nutrition Tip

✳ Shallots, even given the relatively small quantities in which they are included, provide good quantities of vitamin A.

Grilled Bison with Rosemary Marinade

Preparation: 15 minutes ✴ *Cooking: 20 minutes* ✴ *Serves 4*

In addition to the preparation time, you'll need to marinate the bison for at least 4 hours. Because there is not much fatty tissue in bison meat, it's important to marinate the tenderloin before cooking. The marinade tenderizes the meat fibers while adding a distinct, delicious flavor. When substituting beef the nutritional analysis is: calories 135 (kilojoules 565); total fat 2g; saturated fat 1g; protein 25g; cholesterol 70mg; carbohydrates 2g; sodium 206mg; dietary fiber 0g; and calories from fat 15%.

✴ To make the marinade, in a food processor with the metal blade or in a blender, combine the garlic, shallots, parsley, rosemary, broth, soy sauce, lemon juice, lemon zest and peppercorns and process until smooth.

✴ Place the bison or beef in a shallow glass baking dish and pour in the marinade. Cover and refrigerate for 4 hours to 2 days, turning the meat occasionally.

✴ Prepare a fire in an outdoor charcoal grill or preheat a broiler (griller). Place the bison or beef on the grill or in the broiler and discard the marinade. Grill or broil the bison for 10 minutes or beef for 15 minutes. Turn and grill or broil until the meat is medium-rare, 5–10 minutes more.

✴ To serve, slice and divide among 4 individual plates.

Nutritional Analysis per Serving

Calories 132 (Kilojoules 554); Total fat 2g; Saturated fat 1g; Protein 25g;
Cholesterol 70mg; Carbohydrates 2g; Sodium 201mg; Dietary fiber 0g;
Calories from fat 15%

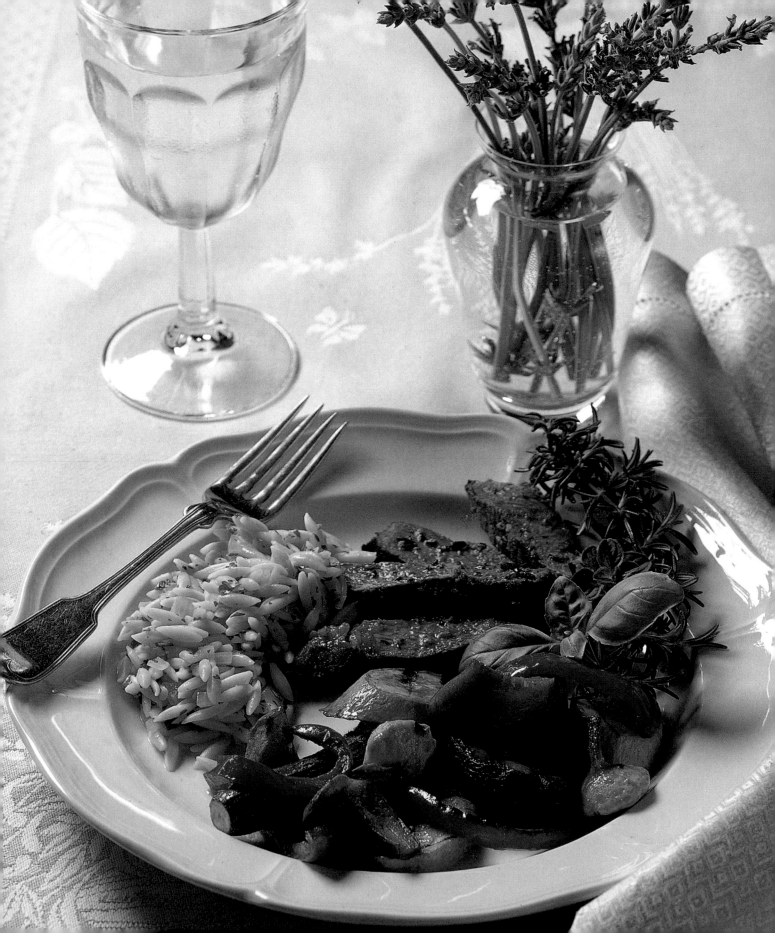

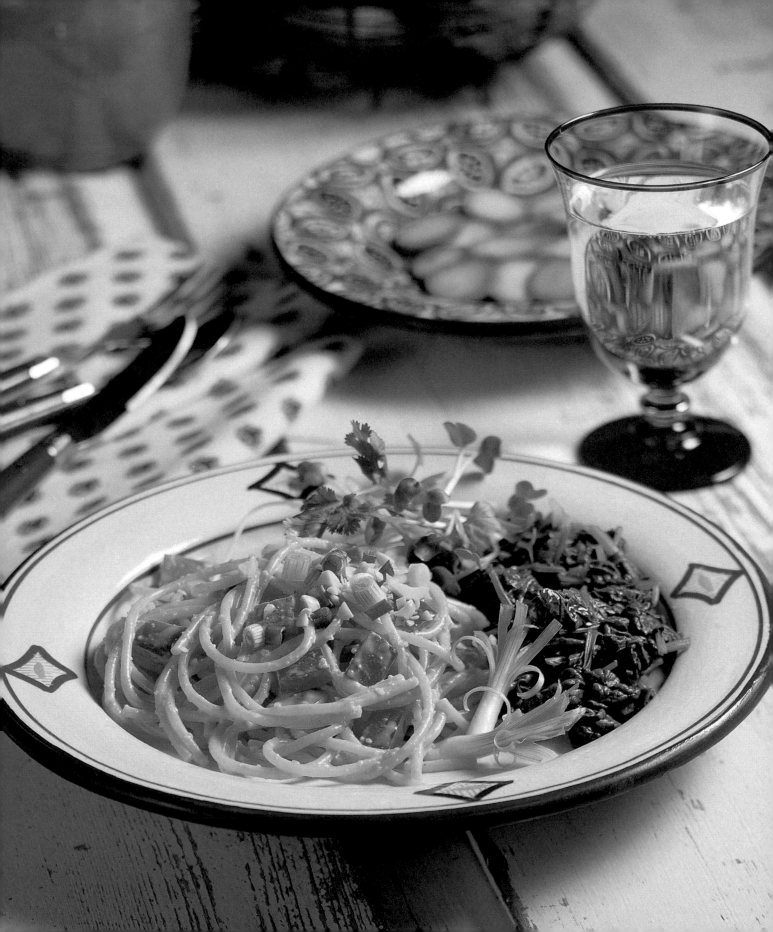

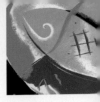

½ cup (4 fl oz/125 ml) Vegetable
Stock (recipe on page 207) or
vegetable broth

3 tablespoons reduced fat chunky
peanut butter

1 tablespoon reduced sodium soy sauce

1 garlic clove, peeled and minced

¼ teaspoon crushed red pepper flakes

6 qt (6 l) water

12 oz (375 g) dried spaghetti

1 green bell pepper (capsicum), seeded,
deribbed and chopped

1 red bell pepper (capsicum), seeded,
deribbed and chopped

½ cup chopped green (spring) onions,
green and white parts

¼ cup (⅓ oz/10 g) chopped fresh
cilantro (fresh coriander)

Cooking Tip

✳ To test that pasta is done al dente, use
a long fork to remove a piece about
1 minute before the allotted cooking time.
Let it cool briefly, then taste. When al
dente it should be tender and cooked
through but still chewy.

Spaghetti in Spicy Peanut Sauce

Preparation: 15 minutes ✳ *Cooking: 10 minutes* ✳ *Serves 4*

*Although peanut butter is high in fat, a little goes a long way in provid-
ing protein, fiber, B vitamins, minerals and an interesting taste to this
vegetarian dish. For the best flavor and texture, purchase pasta made from
semolina (durum wheat flour). Other pasta may be substituted for the
classic round strands of spaghetti. If you choose to use fresh rather than
dried pasta, cook it for about 3 minutes.*

✳ In a small saucepan over medium-high heat, heat the stock or
broth until hot, about 2 minutes.

✳ To make the sauce, in a medium bowl, combine the hot stock
or broth, peanut butter, soy sauce, garlic and red pepper flakes.

✳ In a large pot over high heat, bring the water to a boil. Add the
spaghetti and cook according to the package directions or until
al dente, about 8 minutes. During the last minute of cooking,
add the bell peppers and blanch for 1 minute. Drain.

✳ In a large bowl, combine the pasta and peppers and the sauce
and toss to coat well.

✳ To serve, divide among 4 individual plates. Top each with an
equal amount of the green onions and cilantro.

Nutritional Analysis per Serving

Calories 409 (Kilojoules 1,719); Total fat 6g; Saturated fat 1g; Protein 15g;
Cholesterol 0mg; Carbohydrates 74g; Sodium 221mg; Dietary fiber 3g;
Calories from fat 13%

2 teaspoons olive oil

1 small onion, chopped

2 garlic cloves, peeled and minced

2 tablespoons lemon juice

2 teaspoons finely grated lemon zest

1 cup (7 oz/220 g) uncooked
   Arborio rice

3 cups (24 fl oz/750 ml) Vegetable
   Stock (recipe on page 207) or
   vegetable broth

2 cups (4 oz/125 g) broccoli florets

1 cup (5 oz/155 g) green peas

⅓ cup (1½ oz/45 g) grated Romano
   cheese

¼ cup (⅓ oz/10 g) chopped fresh
   flat-leaf (Italian) parsley

¼ teaspoon ground black pepper

Storage Tip

✳ The risotto can be stored, covered, in the refrigerator for up to 2 days. Reheat in a saucepan over low heat, adding more stock or water as necessary to prevent sticking.

Lemon-Broccoli Risotto

Preparation: 20 minutes ✳ Cooking: 35 minutes ✳ Serves 4

Arborio rice, a short-grained Italian variety found in well-stocked food stores and delicatessens, gives risotto its unique, creamy texture.

✳ In a large nonstick frying pan over medium heat, heat the oil. Add the onion and garlic and sauté until the onion is tender, about 2 minutes. Add the lemon juice, lemon zest and rice and sauté, stirring frequently, until the rice is golden, about 2 minutes.

✳ Add ½ cup (4 fl oz/125 ml) of the stock or broth, reduce the heat to low and simmer until the liquid is absorbed, about 5 minutes. Continue adding the stock or broth, ½ cup (4 fl oz/125 ml) at a time, stirring constantly and waiting until each addition is absorbed before adding the next, about 5 minutes. With the last ½ cup (4 fl oz/125 ml) of stock or broth, add the broccoli and peas. Cook until the liquid is absorbed and the broccoli and peas are tender, about 5 minutes.

✳ Remove from the heat, add the cheese, parsley and pepper and stir until the cheese melts.

✳ To serve, divide among 4 individual plates.

Nutritional Analysis per Serving

Calories 317 (Kilojoules 1,332); Total fat 6g; Saturated fat 0g; Protein 11g; Cholesterol 11mg; Carbohydrates 55g; Sodium 193mg; Dietary fiber 3g; Calories from fat 17%

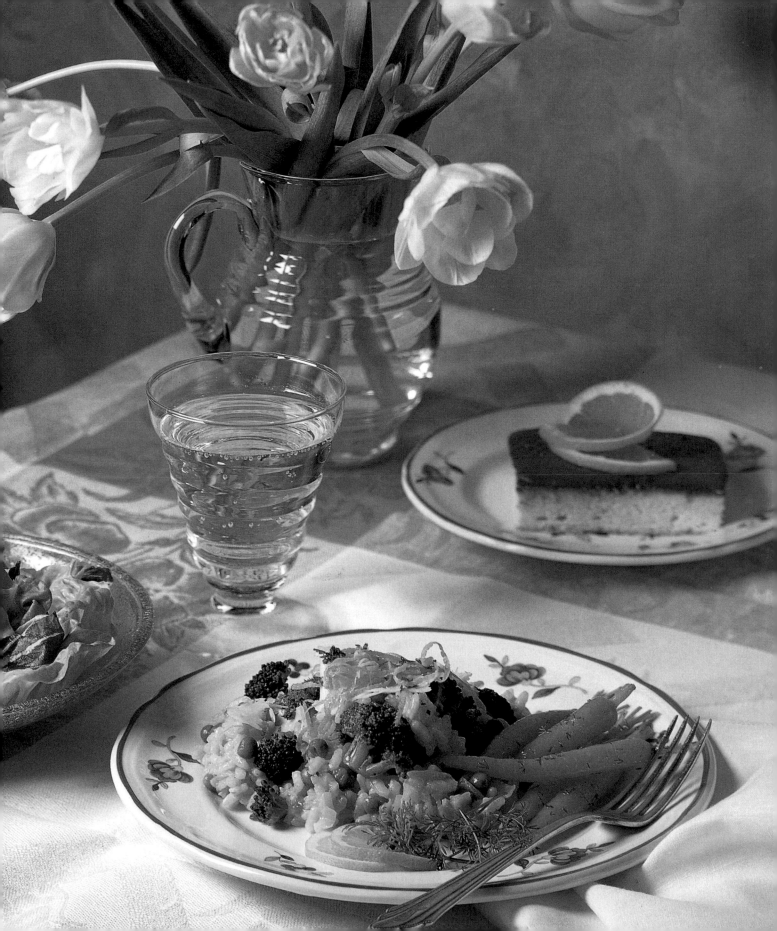

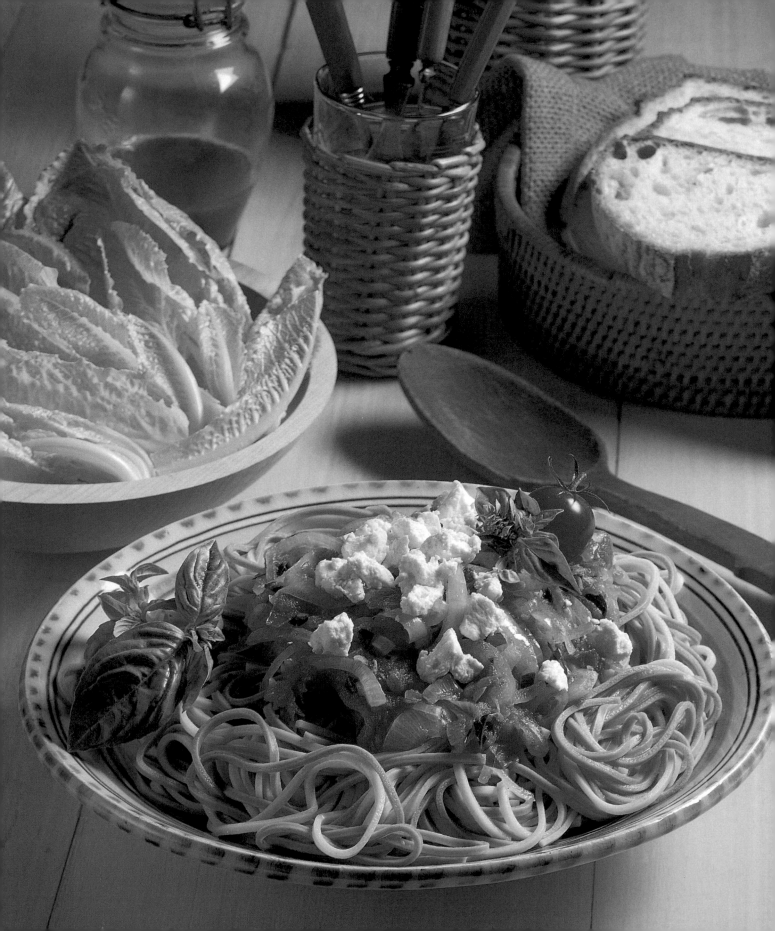

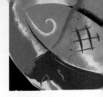

Linguine with Goat Cheese, Tomatoes and Onions

2 teaspoons olive oil

2 onions, thinly sliced

1 tablespoon sugar

2 garlic cloves, peeled, and minced

6 large tomatoes, peeled, seeded
   and chopped

¼ cup (⅓ oz/10 g) chopped fresh basil

2 tablespoons chopped fresh oregano

¼ teaspoon ground black pepper

6 qt (6 l) water

12 oz (375 g) dried linguine

½ cup (2½ oz/75 g) crumbled
   goat cheese

Shopping Tip

✳ When tomatoes are out of season,
substitute about 6 oz (185 g) of canned
diced tomatoes for each large fresh tomato.
Drain off the excess juice from the can
before use.

Preparation: 25 minutes ✳ Cooking: 25 minutes ✳ Serves 4

*The tomatoes give this dish a healthy dose of the antioxidant vitamin C
and, along with the pasta, lots of fiber. Cheese made from goat's milk is
chalky white and available in a variety of shapes and sizes. Young and
fresh versions are mild and creamy; aged cheeses are stronger and drier.
Either can be used to add a tangy taste to this vegetarian pasta dish.*

✳ To make the sauce, in a large nonstick frying pan over medium
heat, heat the oil. Add the onions and sugar and sauté, stirring
frequently, until the onions are golden, about 5 minutes. Add the
garlic and sauté, stirring frequently, for 2 minutes more. Add the
tomatoes, basil, oregano and pepper. Bring to a boil, reduce the
heat to low and simmer until reduced slightly, about 5 minutes.

✳ In a large pot over high heat, bring the water to a boil. Add
the linguine and cook according to the package directions or
until al dente, 8–10 minutes. Drain.

✳ To serve, divide the linguine among 4 individual plates. Top
each with an equal amount of the sauce and goat cheese.

Nutritional Analysis per Serving

Calories 497 (Kilojoules 2,087); Total fat 10g; Saturated fat 4g; Protein 18g;
Cholesterol 14mg; Carbohydrates 86g; Sodium 121mg; Dietary fiber 6g;
Calories from fat 17%

Vegetable Lasagna

*Preparation: 1 hour * Cooking: 1 hour * Serves 6*

No one will miss the meat in this delectable vegetarian version of the classic Italian casserole. Although it is designed as a main dish, you can serve it as a side dish for 12. It's an especially good choice for a buffet supper or to make ahead and have on hand for a last-minute meal.

✻ Preheat an oven to 350°F (180°C). Coat a 13-by-9-inch (33-by-23-cm) baking dish with nonstick cooking spray.

✻ In a medium saucepan over medium heat, combine the onion, tomatoes, basil, thyme and oregano. Bring to a boil, reduce the heat to low and simmer, uncovered, until the sauce has thickened, about 10 minutes. Remove from the heat.

✻ In a food processor with the metal blade or in a blender, combine the garlic, spinach, ricotta, half of the mozzarella, the egg whites, nutmeg and pepper. Process until blended.

✻ In a large pot over high heat, bring the water to a boil. Add the noodles and cook according to the package directions or until al dente, about 10 minutes. Drain.

✻ In the prepared pan, layer 3 noodles, half of the spinach mixture, half of the zucchini and mushroom slices and one-third of the tomato sauce. Repeat the layers, using 3 noodles, the remaining spinach mixture, the remaining zucchini and mushroom slices and half of the remaining tomato sauce. Top with the remaining noodles, the remaining tomato sauce and the remaining mozzarella. Sprinkle with the Romano cheese.

✻ Bake, uncovered, until bubbly and golden on top, about 45 minutes. Cool for 10 minutes before slicing.

✻ To serve, divide among 6 individual plates.

Ingredients

1 onion, chopped

4 large tomatoes, peeled, seeded and chopped

¼ cup (⅓ oz/10 g) chopped fresh basil

2 tablespoons chopped fresh thyme

2 tablespoons chopped fresh oregano

4 garlic cloves, peeled

10 oz (315 g) spinach, stems trimmed

1½ cups (15 oz/375 g) nonfat ricotta cheese

2 cups (8 oz/250 g) grated mozzarella cheese

2 egg whites

½ teaspoon ground nutmeg

¼ teaspoon ground black pepper

6 qt (6 l) water

9 dried lasagna noodles

1 zucchini (courgette), sliced

8 oz (250 g) fresh mushrooms, sliced

2 tablespoons freshly grated Romano cheese

Storage Tip

✻ The casserole can be assembled ahead, covered with plastic wrap or foil and refrigerated for up to 2 days or frozen in an airtight container for up to 1 month. Defrost in the refrigerator before baking.

Nutritional Analysis per Serving

Calories 439 (Kilojoules 1,845); Total fat 8g; Saturated fat 4g; Protein 32g; Cholesterol 24mg; Carbohydrates 58g; Sodium 349mg; Dietary fiber 5g; Calories from fat 17%

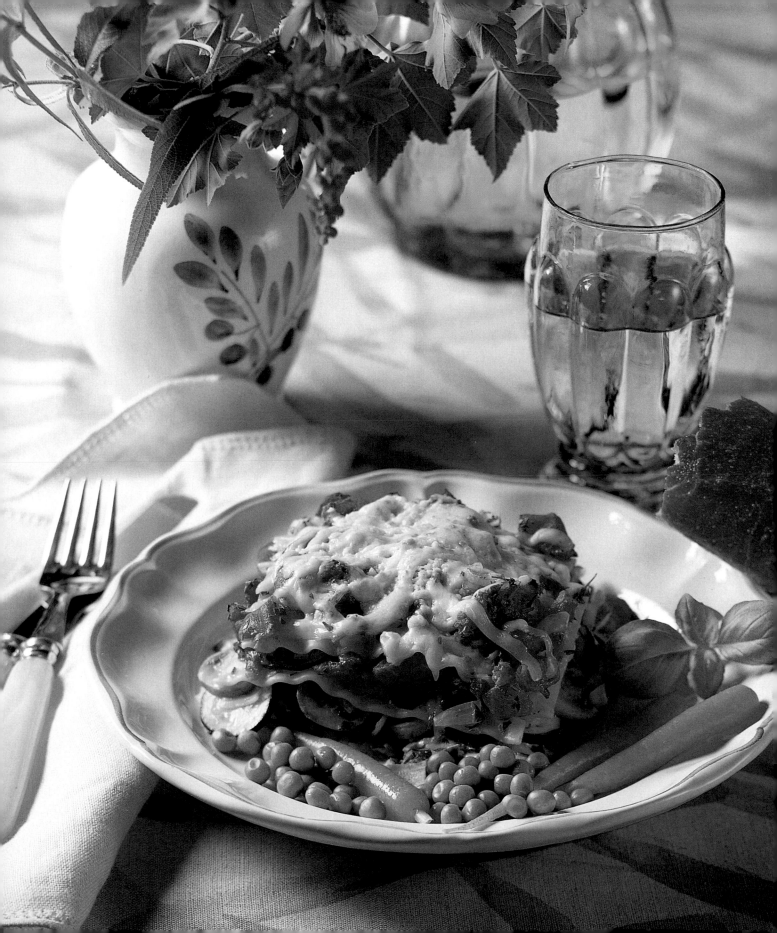

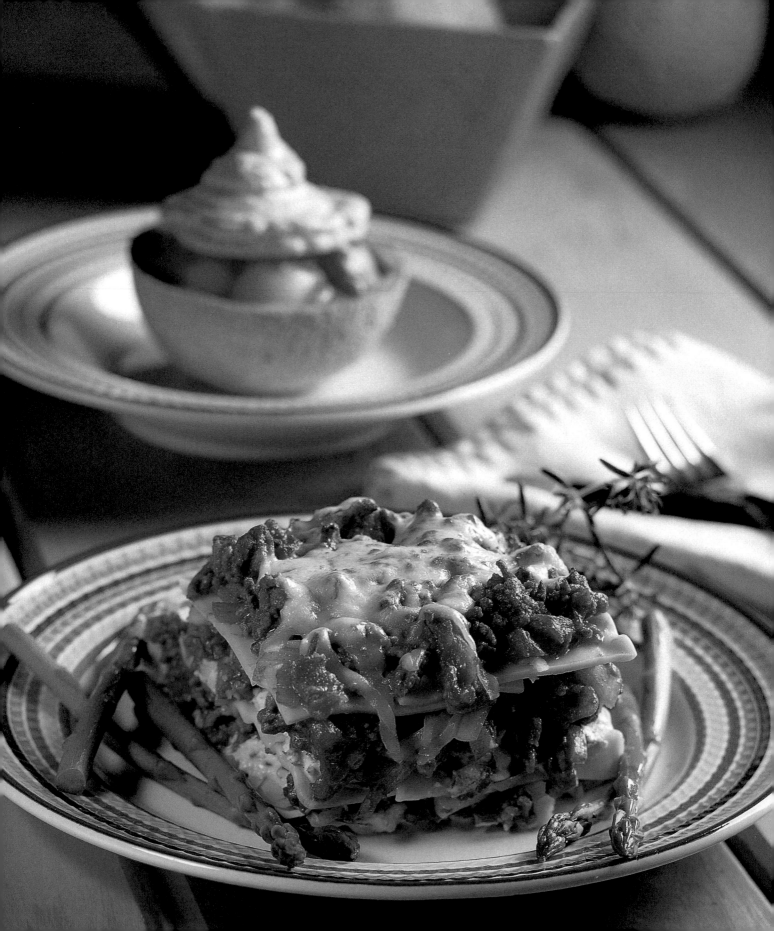

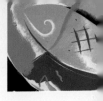

Bison Lasagna

½ lb (250 g) ground bison or ground turkey

1 onion, chopped

8 garlic cloves, peeled and minced

2 large tomatoes, peeled, seeded and chopped

¼ cup (2 fl oz/60 ml) reduced sodium beef broth or beef stock

2 tablespoons chopped fresh oregano

2 tablespoons chopped fresh rosemary

¼ teaspoon ground black pepper

2 cups (16 oz/500 g) nonfat ricotta cheese

1 cup (1½ oz/45 g) chopped fresh basil

½ cup (4 oz/125 g) chopped sun-dried tomatoes, packed without oil

2 tablespoons grated Parmesan cheese

6 qt (6 l) water

9 dried lasagna noodles

1½ cups (6 oz/185 g) grated mozzarella cheese

Preparation: 45 minutes * Cooking: 1 hour 15 minutes * Serves 6

If substituting turkey, the nutritional analysis is: calories 501 (kilojoules 2,103); total fat 7g; saturated fat 4g; protein 39g; cholesterol 41mg; carbohydrates 67g; sodium 357mg; dietary fiber 7g; calories from fat 14%.

✳ Preheat an oven to 350°F (180°C). Coat a 13-by-9-inch (33-by-23-cm) baking dish with nonstick cooking spray.

✳ Coat a large nonstick frying pan with nonstick cooking spray and set over medium heat. Add the bison or turkey, the onion and half of the garlic and sauté until the meat is browned and no longer pink, about 5 minutes. Stir in the chopped tomatoes, broth or stock, oregano, rosemary and pepper. Bring to a boil, reduce the heat to low and simmer, uncovered, until the sauce has thickened, about 10 minutes. Remove from the heat.

✳ In a food processor with the metal blade or in a blender, combine the ricotta cheese, basil, sun-dried tomatoes, Parmesan cheese and remaining garlic. Process until smooth.

✳ In large pot over high heat, bring the water to a boil. Add the noodles and cook according to the package directions or until al dente, about 10 minutes. Drain.

✳ In the prepared pan, layer 3 noodles, half of the ricotta mixture, one-third of the meat sauce and one-third of the mozzarella. Repeat the layers, using 3 noodles, the remaining ricotta mixture, half of the remaining meat sauce and half of the remaining mozzarella. Top with the remaining noodles, the remaining meat sauce and the remaining mozzarella.

✳ Bake, uncovered, until bubbly and golden on top, 35–45 minutes. Cool for 10 minutes before slicing.

✳ To serve, divide among 6 individual plates.

Nutritional Analysis per Serving

Calories 495 (Kilojoules 2,078); Total fat 7g; Saturated fat 4g; Protein 39g; Cholesterol 41mg; Carbohydrates 66g; Sodium 333mg; Dietary fiber 6g; Calories from fat 14%

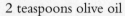

2 teaspoons olive oil

8 garlic cloves, peeled and minced

2 small shallots, peeled and minced

4 large tomatoes, peeled, seeded and
   diced

1 tablespoon chopped fresh oregano

½ teaspoon crushed red pepper flakes

½ teaspoon salt

6 qt (6 l) water

12 oz (375 g) dried penne pasta

¼ cup (⅓ oz/10 g) chopped fresh
   flat-leaf (Italian) parsley

2 tablespoons grated Romano cheese

Cooking Tip

✳ For a dish in the style of pasta primavera, stir steamed fresh vegetables, such as broccoli, asparagus, green peas and bell peppers, into the tomato sauce before spooning over the pasta.

Penne with Garlic-Tomato Sauce

Preparation: 15 minutes ✳ Cooking: 30 minutes ✳ Serves 4

I always ask that this sauce recipe be doubled or tripled and put into jars in the refrigerator so that I can use it to top pasta, rice, polenta or even potatoes as a very quick late-night supper.

✳ In a large nonstick frying pan over medium heat, heat the oil. Add the garlic and shallots and sauté until tender, about 3 minutes.

✳ Add the tomatoes and oregano, bring to a boil, reduce the heat to low and simmer for 10 minutes. Add the red pepper flakes and salt and simmer for 5 minutes more. Keep warm.

✳ In a large pot over high heat, bring the water to a boil. Add the penne and cook according to the package directions or until al dente, 8–10 minutes. Drain. Add the penne to the frying pan and stir to coat well.

✳ To serve, divide among 4 individual plates. Top each with an equal amount of the parsley and cheese.

Nutritional Analysis per Serving

Calories 386 (Kilojoules 1,623); Total fat 5g; Saturated fat 1g; Protein 13g; Cholesterol 3mg; Carbohydrates 73g; Sodium 325mg; Dietary fiber 4g; Calories from fat 11%

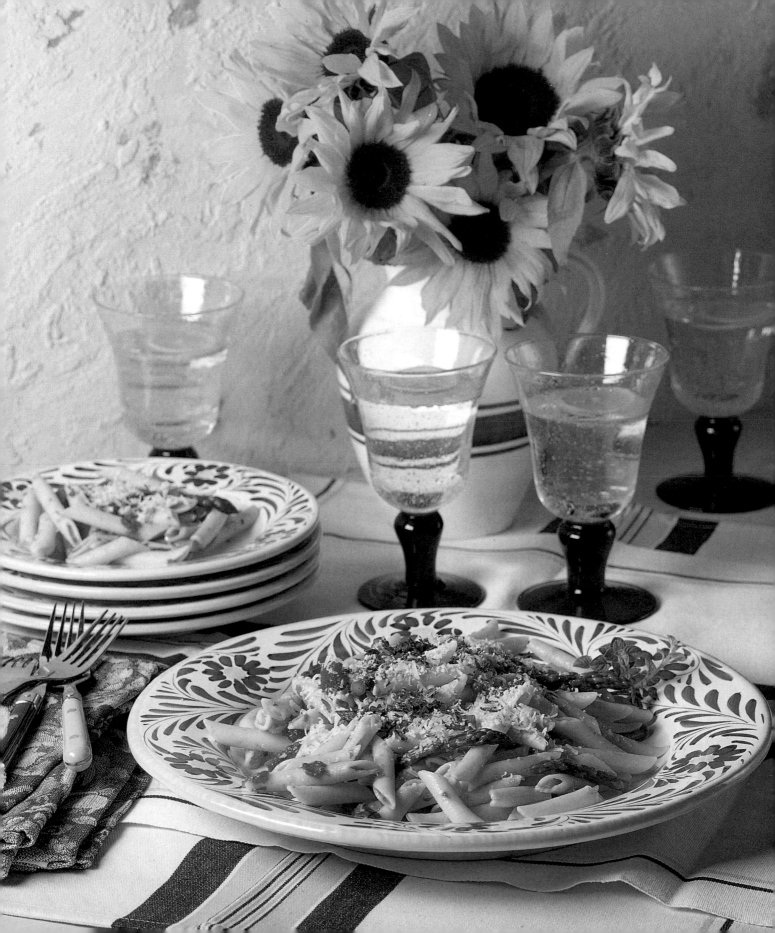

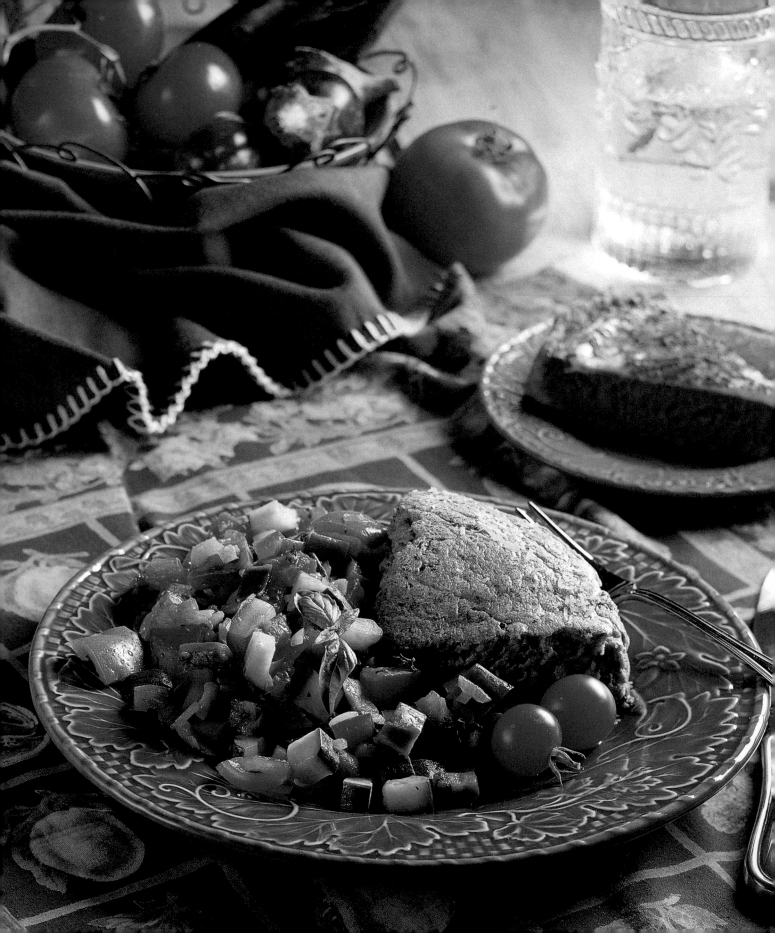

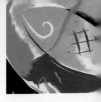

1 tablespoon grated Parmesan cheese

12 oz (375 g) spinach, stems trimmed

2 shallots, peeled and halved

2½ tablespoons margarine

¼ cup (1½ oz/45 g) unbleached flour

1½ cups (12 fl oz/375 ml) nonfat milk

6 egg whites

¼ teaspoon cream of tartar

1 cup (4 oz/125 g) grated lowfat
   Swiss cheese

1 teaspoon chili powder

¼ teaspoon ground nutmeg

Cooking Tip

✻ Although shallots resemble garlic cloves in size and shape, they may be easily peeled for slicing and chopping like an onion. Simply trim off their stem and root ends, then slit their thin papery skins to remove them.

Spinach Soufflé

Preparation: 30 minutes ✻ Cooking: 35 minutes ✻ Serves 4

This soufflé, rich in iron and beta-carotene, is my absolute favorite; it pairs very nicely with the hearty Ratatouille (recipe on page 198). Serve soufflés immediately after removing from the oven as the puff collapses upon cooling.

✻ Preheat an oven to 375°F (190°C). Coat a 2-qt (2-l) soufflé dish with nonstick cooking spray.

✻ Sprinkle the Parmesan cheese into the dish and turn to coat the bottom and sides. Place the dish on a large baking sheet.

✻ In a steaming basket in a saucepan filled with 1 inch (2.5 cm) of water over medium heat, steam the spinach until tender, about 3 minutes. Remove from the basket; squeeze to remove all liquid.

✻ In a food processor with the metal blade or in a blender, combine the spinach and shallots and process until finely chopped.

✻ In a large nonstick frying pan over low heat, melt the margarine. Add the flour and stir constantly with a wire whisk until blended, about 2 minutes. Increase the heat to medium and gradually add the milk, stirring constantly with a wire whisk, and cook until the mixture boils, about 5 minutes.

✻ Reduce the heat to low, add the spinach mixture and cook until the mixture begins to simmer, about 3 minutes.

✻ In a large bowl, using an electric mixer on high speed, beat the egg whites until foamy. Add the cream of tartar and beat on high speed until stiff peaks form.

✻ In a large bowl, combine one-fourth of the egg whites, the Swiss cheese, chili powder, nutmeg and the spinach mixture and whisk to mix well. Fold in the remaining egg whites. Pour into the prepared dish and bake until puffed and set, 30–35 minutes.

✻ To serve, divide among 4 individual plates.

Nutritional Analysis per Serving

Calories 284 (Kilojoules 1,194); Total fat 14g; Saturated fat 2g; Protein 19g; Cholesterol 12mg; Carbohydrates 17g; Sodium 418mg; Dietary fiber 3g; Calories from fat 47%

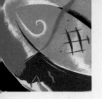

1 cup (7 oz/220 g) dried black beans

4 cups (32 fl oz/1 l) water

2 teaspoons olive oil

1 large onion, chopped

3 garlic cloves, peeled and minced

1½ teaspoons chili powder

1 teaspoon ground cumin

2 large tomatoes, peeled, seeded and
    chopped

1 cup (6 oz/185 g) corn kernels

3 jalapeño chilies, seeded and
    chopped

¼ teaspoon salt

¼ teaspoon ground black pepper

8 corn tortillas, 6 inches (15 cm) in
    diameter

½ cup (4 oz/125 g) nonfat dairy
    sour cream

½ cup (2 oz/60 g) grated lowfat
    Monterey jack cheese

Tomato Salsa

2 tomatoes, seeded and chopped

⅓ cup (1 oz/30 g) chopped red onion

1 jalapeño chili, seeded and diced

1 tablespoon chopped fresh cilantro
    (fresh coriander)

1 teaspoon lime juice

⅛ teaspoon salt

⅛ teaspoon ground black pepper

Black Bean Enchiladas with Tomato Salsa

*Preparation: 20 minutes * Cooking: 2 hours * Serves 4*

Pair this vegetarian main dish with rice, as combined portions of beans and rice provide the complete protein but none of the fat of a meat-based meal.

✴ In a large saucepan over high heat, combine the beans and water and bring to a boil. Reduce the heat to medium and cook for 1½ hours, skimming away the gray foam that appears. Drain well.

✴ Preheat an oven to 350°F (180°C). Coat a 13-by-9-inch (33-by-23-cm) baking dish with nonstick cooking spray.

✴ In a large nonstick frying pan over medium heat, heat the oil. Add the onion and garlic and sauté for 3 minutes. Add the chili powder and cumin and sauté for 1 minute. Add half of the tomatoes and the corn, chilies, salt and pepper and simmer for 1 minute.

✴ Wrap the tortillas in aluminum foil and warm in the oven for 5 minutes.

✴ In a food processor with the metal blade, combine the beans and sour cream and process until smooth. Add to the frying pan and cook until the beans are warm, about 3 minutes.

✴ Divide the bean mixture among the tortillas. Roll and place seam side down in the prepared dish. Top with the remaining tomatoes and the cheese. Cover with aluminum foil and bake until the cheese melts, about 20 minutes.

✴ To serve, divide among 4 individual plates. Top each with an equal amount of the Tomato Salsa.

Tomato Salsa

✴ In a medium bowl, combine the tomatoes, onion, chili, cilantro, lime juice, salt and pepper. Stir to mix well. Cover and refrigerate until serving. One serving is ½ cup (3 oz/90 g).

Nutritional Analysis per Serving

Calories 465 (Kilojoules 1,954); Total fat 8g; Saturated fat 3g; Protein 24g; Cholesterol 10mg; Carbohydrates 79g; Sodium 451mg; Dietary fiber 14g; Calories from fat 15%

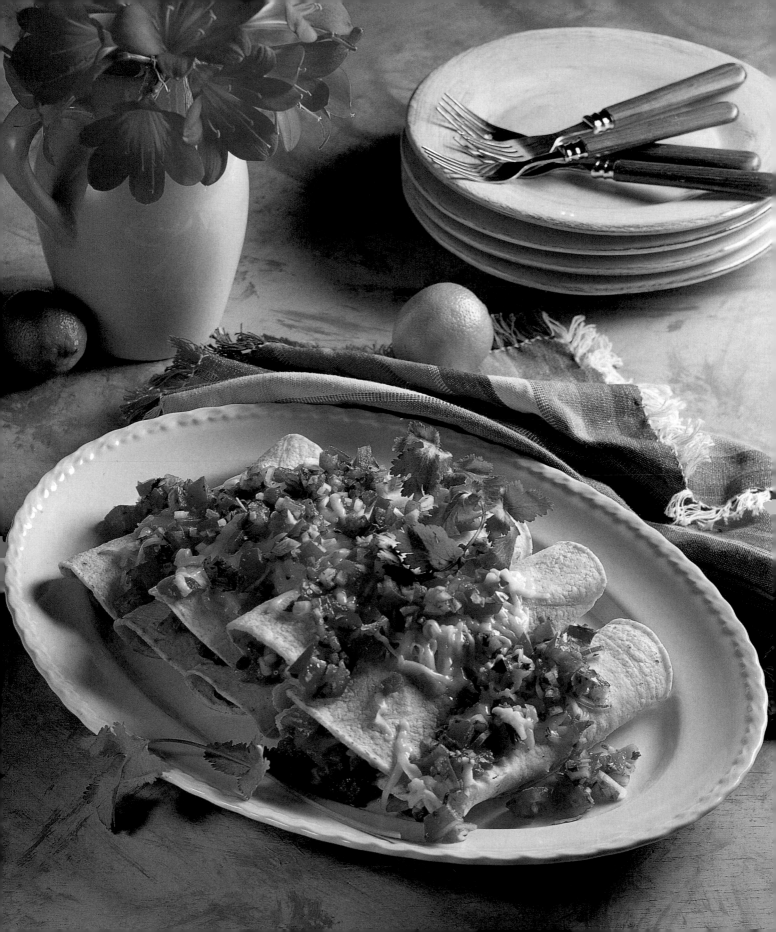

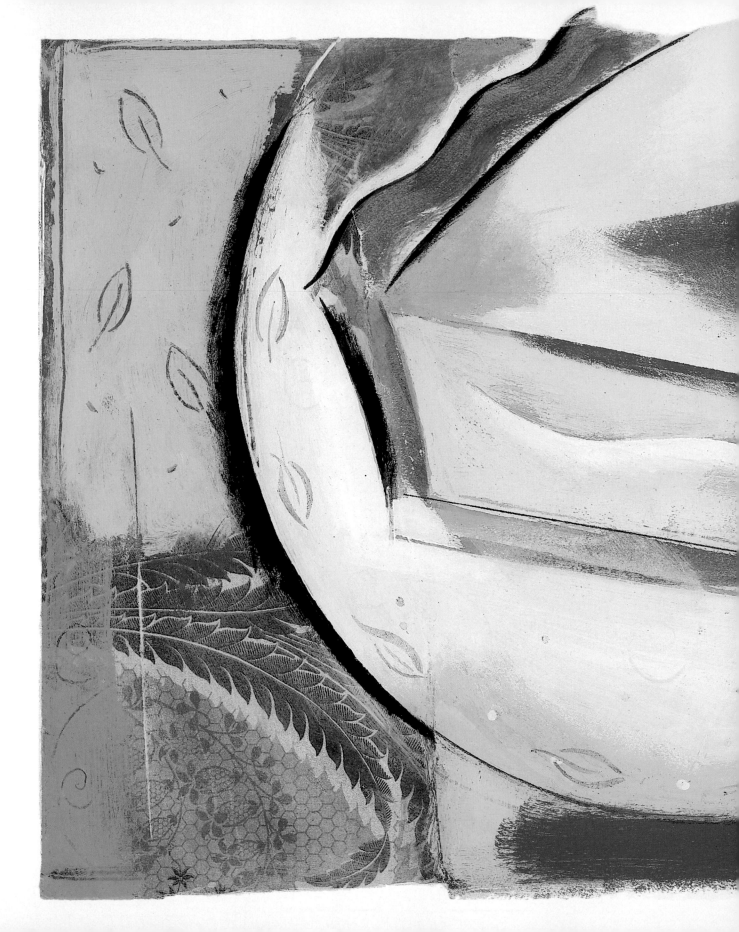

Completing the Meal

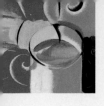

2 cups (8 oz/250 g) strawberries, stemmed and cored

2 bananas, peeled

1½ cups (12 fl oz/375 ml) cranberry juice

1 cup (8 oz/250 g) crushed ice

Strawberry-Banana Shake

Preparation: 10 minutes ✳ Serves 4

Shakes and smoothies are my morning drink of choice. This sweet-tart version is packed with fresh-fruit goodness. If you haven't already, add cranberry juice to your juice repertoire. It is an ample source of vitamin C and aids in flushing toxins from the body.

✳ In a food processor with the metal blade or in a blender, combine the strawberries, bananas and cranberry juice and process until smooth. Add the crushed ice and process until smooth.

✳ To serve, divide among 4 individual glasses.

Nutritional Analysis per Serving

Calories 123 (Kilojoules 519); Total fat 1g; Saturated fat 0g; Protein 1g; Cholesterol 0mg; Carbohydrates 31g; Sodium 3mg; Dietary fiber 2g; Calories from fat 4%

1 cup (8 oz/250 g) orange sherbet or frozen yogurt

1 cup (4 oz/125 g) strawberries, stemmed and cored

1⅓ cups (8 oz/250 g) pineapple chunks

1½ cups (12 fl oz/375 ml) sparkling mineral water

Sunshine Smoothie

Preparation: 10 minutes ✳ Serves 4

As the name implies, this smoothie gets your day off to a sunny start, fulfilling 2 fruit servings of your recommended daily food requirements before you've left the house. If you're in a hurry and must eat on the run, take this healthy breakfast drink in an insulated car cup to drink while you drive.

✳ In a food processor with the metal blade or in a blender, combine the sherbet or yogurt, strawberries and pineapple and process until smooth. Add the water and process until blended.

✳ To serve, divide among 4 individual glasses.

Nutritional Analysis per Serving

Calories 115 (Kilojoules 481); Total fat 1g; Saturated fat 1g; Protein 1g; Cholesterol 3mg; Carbohydrates 26g; Sodium 27mg; Dietary fiber 1g; Calories from fat 11%

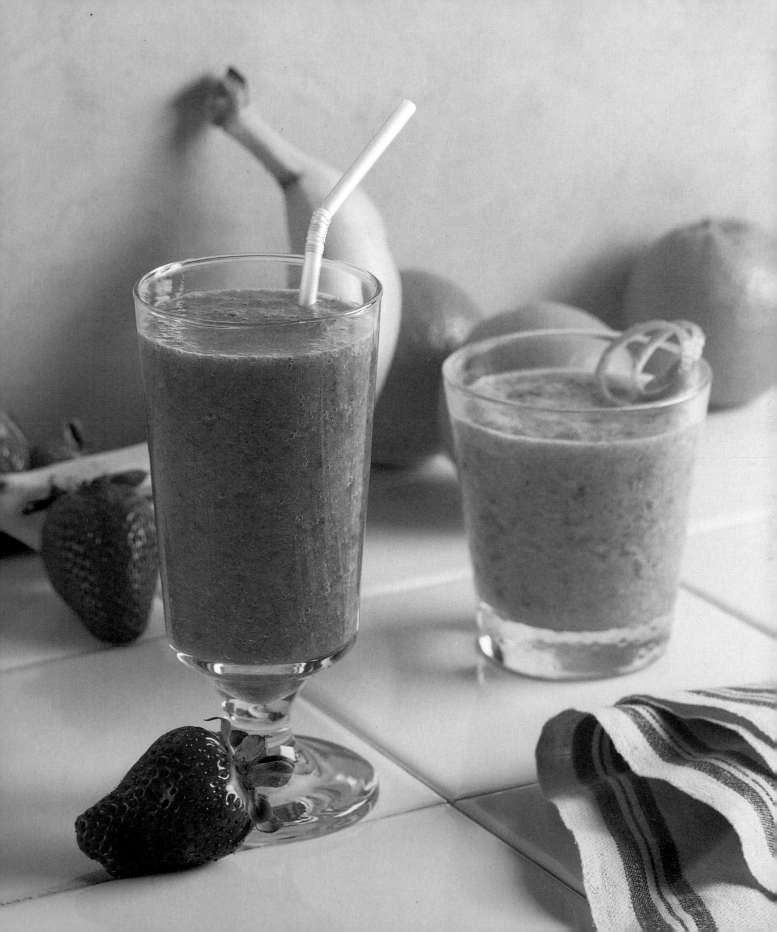

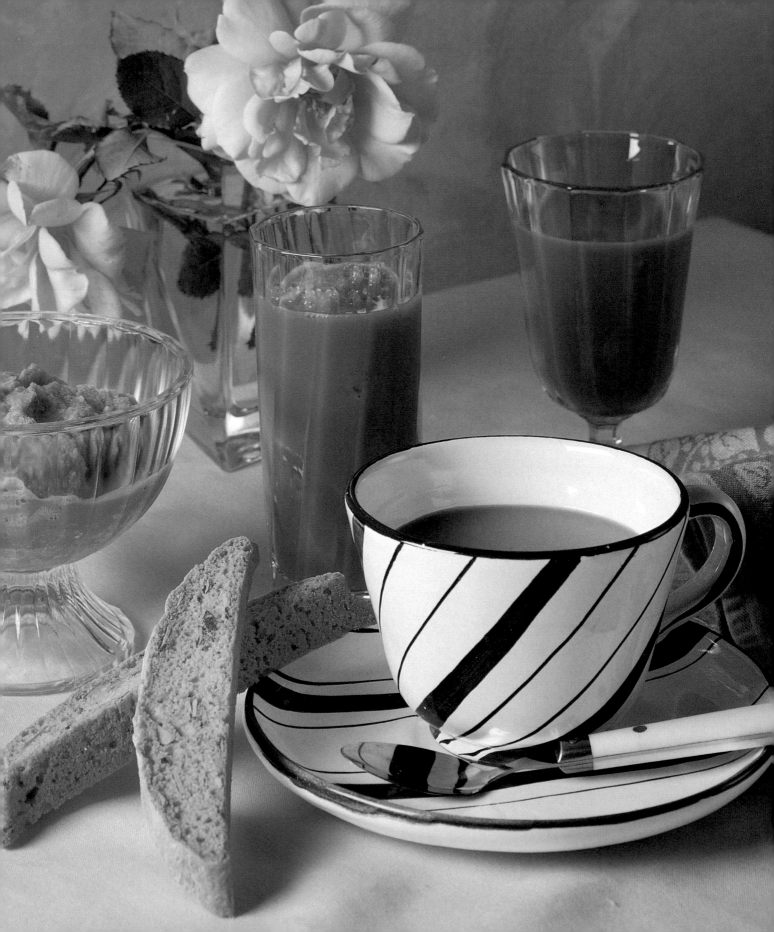

4 cups (32 fl oz/1 l) nonfat milk

3 tablespoons sugar

4 teaspoons unsweetened Dutch-
process cocoa

1 teaspoon vanilla extract (essence)

Iced Cocoa

✳ For a lowfat chocolate dessert, freeze the Hot Cocoa. When the mixture is firm, process in a food processor with the metal blade or in a blender until smooth. To serve, spoon into dessert bowls.

Hot Cocoa

Preparation: 5 minutes ✳ *Serves 4*

It is hard to believe—but true—that one serving of this cocoa contains just 1 g of fat. Serve it piping hot as a breakfast beverage or iced as a dessert (recipe at left).

✳ In a small saucepan over medium heat, warm the milk until bubbles just begin to appear around the edge, about 5 minutes. Gradually add the sugar, cocoa and vanilla and whisk until dissolved and blended.

✳ To serve, divide among 4 individual mugs.

Nutritional Analysis per Serving

Calories 130 (Kilojoules 548); Total fat 1g; Saturated fat 0g; Protein 9g; Cholesterol 5mg; Carbohydrates 22g; Sodium 140mg; Dietary fiber 0g; Calories from fat 5%

---

4 cups (32 fl oz/1 l) strong, freshly brewed coffee

1 cup (8 fl oz/250 ml) lowfat (1%) milk

4 tablespoons confectioners' (icing) sugar

2 tablespoons unsweetened Dutch-
process cocoa

1 teaspoon vanilla extract (essence)

Iced Skinny Café Mocha

✳ For a refreshingly cool drink, pour the Skinny Café Mocha into a heatproof glass container and cool. Cover and refrigerate for 4 hours. To serve, spoon shaved ice into tall glasses. Top with the chilled coffee.

Skinny Café Mocha

Preparation: 15 minutes ✳ *Serves 4*

Fancy coffee bars serve lowfat versions of their mocha-flavored coffees and now you can, too. On a hot afternoon, the iced version (recipe at left) will clear your head and give you an energy boost.

✳ In a medium saucepan over low heat, combine the coffee, milk, sugar and cocoa. Simmer until the sugar is dissolved, about 5 minutes. Remove from the heat and stir in the vanilla.

✳ To serve, divide among 4 individual mugs.

Nutritional Analysis per Serving

Calories 70 (Kilojoules 295); Total fat 1g; Saturated fat 1g; Protein 3g; Cholesterol 2mg; Carbohydrates 13g; Sodium 55mg; Dietary fiber 0g; Calories from fat 14%

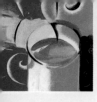

Tangy Tomato Drink

4 cups (32 fl oz/1 l) low sodium
   tomato juice
2 tablespoons lemon juice
1½ teaspoons Worcestershire sauce
½ teaspoon ground celery seed
1 teaspoon drained, grated horseradish
¼ teaspoon ground black pepper
4 celery stalks
1 tablespoon chopped fresh flat-leaf
   (Italian) parsley

*Preparation: 15 minutes * Serves 4*

Mixing your own tomato juice cocktail allows you to control what's in it. Many similar commercial drinks are loaded with salt, MSG and other additives. The health benefits derived from this version outweigh the few moments it takes to put together.

✳ In a large pitcher, combine the tomato juice, lemon juice, Worcestershire sauce, celery seed, horseradish and pepper. Stir to mix well.

✳ To serve, divide among 4 individual glasses. Garnish each with a celery stalk and an equal amount of the parsley.

Nutritional Analysis per Serving

Calories 53 (Kilojoules 225); Total fat 0g; Saturated fat 0g; Protein 2g; Cholesterol 0mg; Carbohydrates 13g; Sodium 83mg; Dietary fiber 1g; Calories from fat 4%

Hot Fruit Cider

4 cups (32 fl oz/1 l) apple cider
1 tart apple, peeled, cored and sliced
2 lemon slices
1 vanilla bean (pod), 1 inch
   (2.5 cm) long
5 whole cloves
4 whole cinnamon sticks

*Preparation: 10 minutes * Cooking: 10 minutes * Serves 4*

Cider is available with and without alcohol. If possible, use cider made from organic apples. The taste is sensational. You can substitute apple juice, although the flavor will be somewhat less fruity.

✳ In a medium saucepan over medium heat, combine the cider, apple slices, lemon slices, vanilla bean and cloves. Bring to a boil, reduce the heat to low, cover and simmer for 10 minutes. Remove from the heat and strain to remove the solids.

✳ To serve, divide among 4 individual mugs. Garnish each with a cinnamon stick.

Nutritional Analysis per Serving

Calories 138 (Kilojoules 581); Total fat 0g; Saturated fat 0g; Protein 0g; Cholesterol 0mg; Carbohydrates 35g; Sodium 8mg; Dietary fiber 1g; Calories from fat 2%

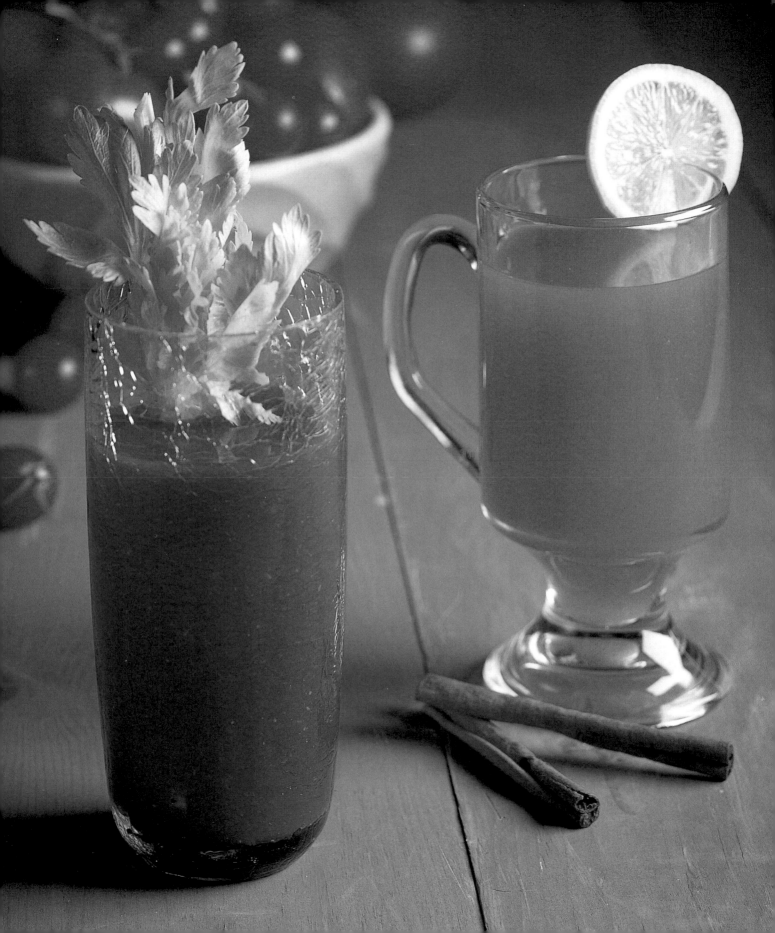

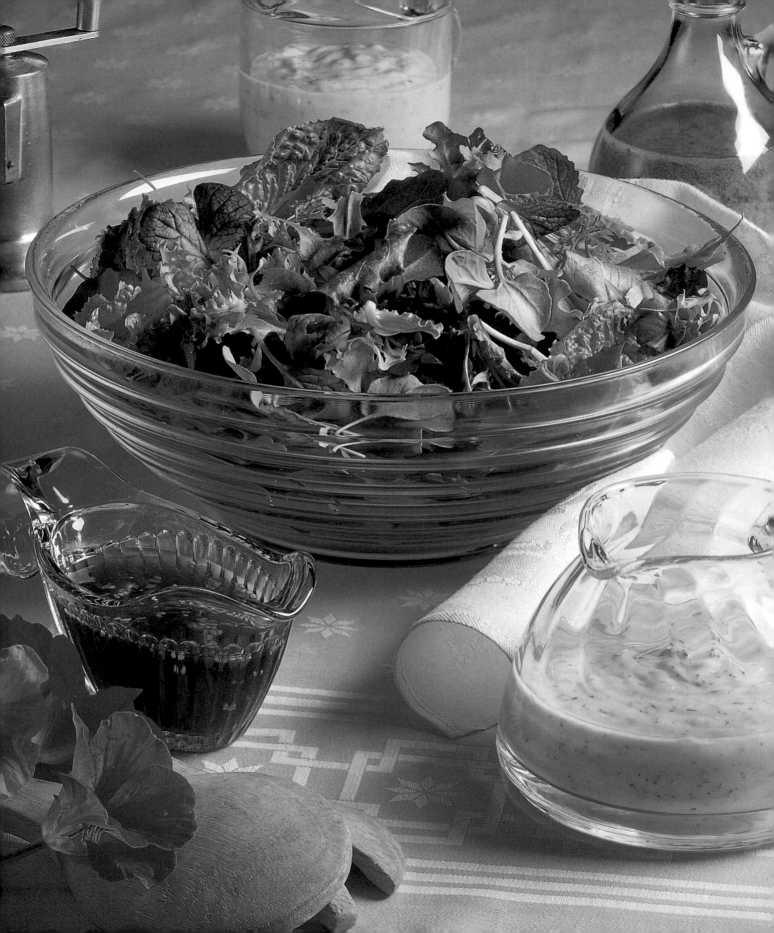

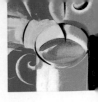

Salad Greens

An abundant range of greens exists to add wide variety to your salad bowls: lettuces, including tender butter lettuces (such as Boston, Bibb and limestone), crisp romaine (cos), and red leaf or oak leaf; chicory (curly endive), with its bitter edge; dark-green, peppery arugula (rocket); refreshingly bitter Belgian endive; crisp, bitter, deep-purple radicchio; and familiar spinach, watercress and cabbages. Seek them out at a well-stocked food store or greengrocer. Separate, wash and dry thoroughly before refrigerating. The dressings shown at left are listed below and on page 184.

Dill Dressing

1 cup (8 oz/250 g) nonfat plain yogurt
¼ cup (⅓ oz/10 g) chopped fresh dill
2 teaspoons red wine vinegar
¼ teaspoon ground black pepper

*Preparation: 10 minutes * Serves 8*

✳ In a small bowl, combine the yogurt, dill, vinegar and pepper and whisk until blended.

✳ Store in an airtight container in the refrigerator for up to 3 days. One serving is 2 tablespoons.

Nutritional Analysis per Serving

Calories 17 (Kilojoules 72); Total fat 0g; Saturated fat 0g; Protein 2g; Cholesterol 1mg; Carbohydrates 2g; Sodium 22mg; Dietary fiber 0g; Calories from fat 3%

Basil Dressing

½ cup (4 fl oz/125 ml) lowfat
   buttermilk
½ cup (4 oz/125 g) nonfat dairy
   sour cream
¼ cup (⅓ oz/10 g) chopped fresh basil
2 teaspoons white wine vinegar
⅛ teaspoon ground white pepper
⅛ teaspoon cayenne pepper

*Preparation: 10 minutes * Serves 8*

✳ In a small bowl, combine the buttermilk, sour cream, basil, vinegar, pepper and cayenne and whisk until blended. Cover and refrigerate until ready to serve. Store in an airtight container in the refrigerator for up to 3 days. One serving is 2 tablespoons.

Nutritional Analysis per Serving

Calories 19 (Kilojoules 81); Total fat 0g; Saturated fat 0g; Protein 2g; Cholesterol 1mg; Carbohydrates 2g; Sodium 32mg; Dietary fiber 0g; Calories from fat 9%

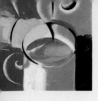

½ cup (4 fl oz/125 ml) rice vinegar

2 tablespoons reduced sodium
soy sauce

2 tablespoons sesame seeds,
lightly toasted

1 teaspoon dark sesame oil

1 garlic clove, peeled and minced

½ teaspoon grated fresh ginger

Cooking Tip

To toast sesame seeds, spread on a baking sheet and bake in a preheated 350°F (180°C) oven, stirring occasionally, until golden, about 5 minutes.

1 teaspoon sugar

½ cup (4 fl oz/125 ml) red
wine vinegar

2 tablespoons Dijon-style mustard

2 tablespoons chopped fresh flat-leaf
(Italian) parsley

1 tablespoon olive oil

1 tablespoon water

¼ teaspoon ground black pepper

Nutrition Tip

✱ The greatest source of fat in many salads comes from the dressing. To get the most flavor but the least fat in your salad, serve the dressing on the side, dipping your fork into it before skewering the greens.

Sesame-Garlic Dressing

Preparation: 10 minutes ✱ *Serves 8*

This Asian-influenced dressing is rich with the taste of sesame. Toasting the sesame seeds brings out their nutty flavor.

✱ In a small bowl, combine the vinegar, soy sauce, sesame seeds, sesame oil, garlic and ginger and whisk until blended.

✱ Cover and refrigerate until ready to serve. Store in an airtight container in the refrigerator for up to 3 days. One serving is 2 tablespoons.

Nutritional Analysis per Serving

Calories 23 (Kilojoules 96); Total fat 2g; Saturated fat 0g; Protein 1g; Cholesterol 0mg; Carbohydrates 2g; Sodium 150mg; Dietary fiber 0g; Calories from fat 63%

Mustard Vinaigrette

Preparation: 10 minutes ✱ *Serves 12*

The Dijon-style mustard, whether made in Dijon, France, or made in the style of that region, is a pale yellow condiment made from a mixture of black or brown mustard seeds, white wine, vinegar, water and salt. It adds zest to this simple vinaigrette.

✱ In a small bowl, dissolve the sugar in the vinegar. Add the mustard, parsley, olive oil, water and pepper and whisk until blended.

✱ Cover and refrigerate until ready to serve. Store in an airtight container in the refrigerator for up to 2 weeks. One serving is 1 tablespoon.

Nutritional Analysis per Serving

Calories 15 (Kilojoules 65); Total fat 1g; Saturated fat 0g; Protein 0g; Cholesterol 0mg; Carbohydrates 1g; Sodium 60mg; Dietary fiber 0g; Calories from fat 77%

1 teaspoon honey

1 cup (8 fl oz/250 ml) lukewarm
  water

2 teaspoons active dry yeast

2 tablespoons olive oil

1 teaspoon salt

1½ cups (7½ oz/235 g) semolina
  flour

1½ cups (7½ oz/235 g) whole wheat
  (wholemeal) flour

Storage Tip

✳ This dough can be made ahead and
frozen for up to 2 months. After the first
rising, wrap in plastic wrap and aluminum
foil and place in the freezer. Thaw at room
temperature and follow the directions
from the second kneading.

Karen's Pizza Dough

Preparation: 25 minutes ✳ *Makes 1 lb (500 g)*

*In addition to the preparation time, allow 1½ hours for the dough to rise.
This dough is easy to work with and tastes just great. Use it as a base
for the pizzas beginning on page 107 or for your own creative versions.*

✳ In a food processor with the metal blade or in a large bowl,
combine the honey and water. Add the yeast to the water and let
stand 5 minutes. Add the oil, salt and flours and process or stir
until the mixture forms a ball, about 30 seconds by machine or
5 minutes by hand.

✳ Turn onto a lightly floured work surface and knead until the
dough is smooth and elastic, about 5 minutes.

✳ Coat a large bowl with nonstick cooking spray, add the dough
and turn to coat all sides. Cover with plastic wrap and let rise in a
warm place, free from draft, until doubled in bulk, about 1 hour.

✳ Return to the lightly floured work surface and using your fist,
punch down the dough, then knead for 2 minutes. Return to the
bowl, cover with plastic wrap and let rise again for 30 minutes.

✳ Use the dough according to recipe instructions. One serving
is ¼ pound (125 g).

Nutritional Analysis per Serving

Calories 458 (Kilojoules 1,926); Total fat 9g; Saturated fat 1g; Protein 15g;
Cholesterol 0mg; Carbohydrates 82g; Sodium 554mg; Dietary fiber 9g;
Calories from fat 17%

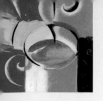

¾ lb (375 g) fresh spinach, stems removed and leaves chopped

1 cup (8 oz/250 g) nonfat cottage cheese

½ cup (4 oz/125 g) nonfat dairy sour cream

1 tablespoon chopped fresh flat-leaf (Italian) parsley

2 shallots, peeled and minced

¼ teaspoon salt

¼ teaspoon ground white pepper

1 cup (8 oz/250 g) sliced water chestnuts

8 oz (250 g) nonfat cream cheese

1 cup (8 oz/250 g) nonfat cottage cheese

⅓ cup (3 oz/90 g) mango chutney

¼ cup (⅓ oz/10 g) chopped fresh flat-leaf (Italian) parsley

2 tablespoons minced fresh chives

2 teaspoons Dijon-style mustard

¼ teaspoon ground black pepper

⅛ teaspoon cayenne pepper

Creamy Spinach Spread

*Preparation: 10 minutes * Serves 12*

Serve this dip on French bread or with fresh vegetables like cherry tomatoes, carrot and celery sticks, cucumber slices, zucchini slices and broccoli and cauliflower florets.

✳ In a food processor with the metal blade or in a blender, combine the spinach, cottage cheese, sour cream, parsley, shallots, salt and pepper. Process until almost smooth. Transfer to a large bowl, add the water chestnuts and stir to mix well.

✳ Store in an airtight container in the refrigerator for up to 3 days. One serving is 2 tablespoons.

Nutritional Analysis per Serving

Calories 48 (Kilojoules 200); Total fat 0g; Saturated fat 0g; Protein 4g; Cholesterol 2mg; Carbohydrates 7g; Sodium 138mg; Dietary fiber 1g; Calories from fat 2%

Chive-Chutney Dip

*Preparation: 10 minutes * Serves 8*

If you are having trouble finding healthy, tasty snacks, your search is over. Make this nonfat herb-fruit dip and keep it in the refrigerator ready to enjoy with peeled and sliced carrots, celery, cucumbers and other vegetables.

✳ In a food processor with the metal blade or in a blender, combine the cream cheese, cottage cheese, chutney, parsley, chives, mustard, black pepper and cayenne. Process until smooth.

✳ Transfer the dip to a serving bowl, cover and refrigerate until ready to serve. Store in the refrigerator for up to 1 week. One serving is ¼ cup (2 oz/60 g).

Nutritional Analysis per Serving

Calories 76 (Kilojoules 319); Total fat 0g; Saturated fat 0g; Protein 8g; Cholesterol 5mg; Carbohydrates 10g; Sodium 360mg; Dietary fiber 0g; Calories from fat 0%

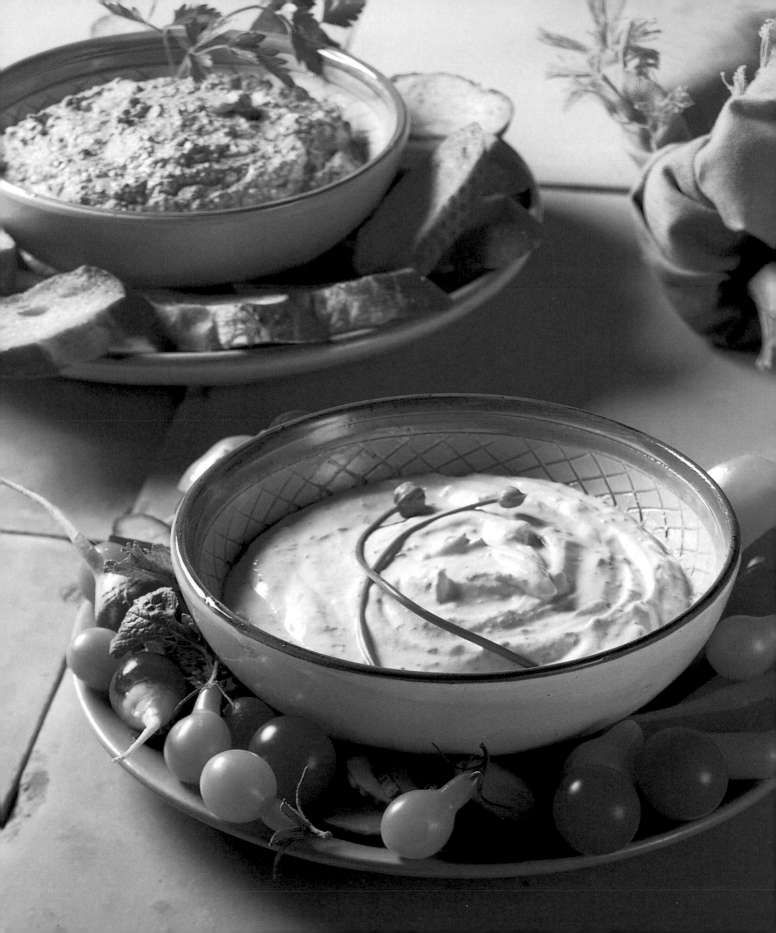

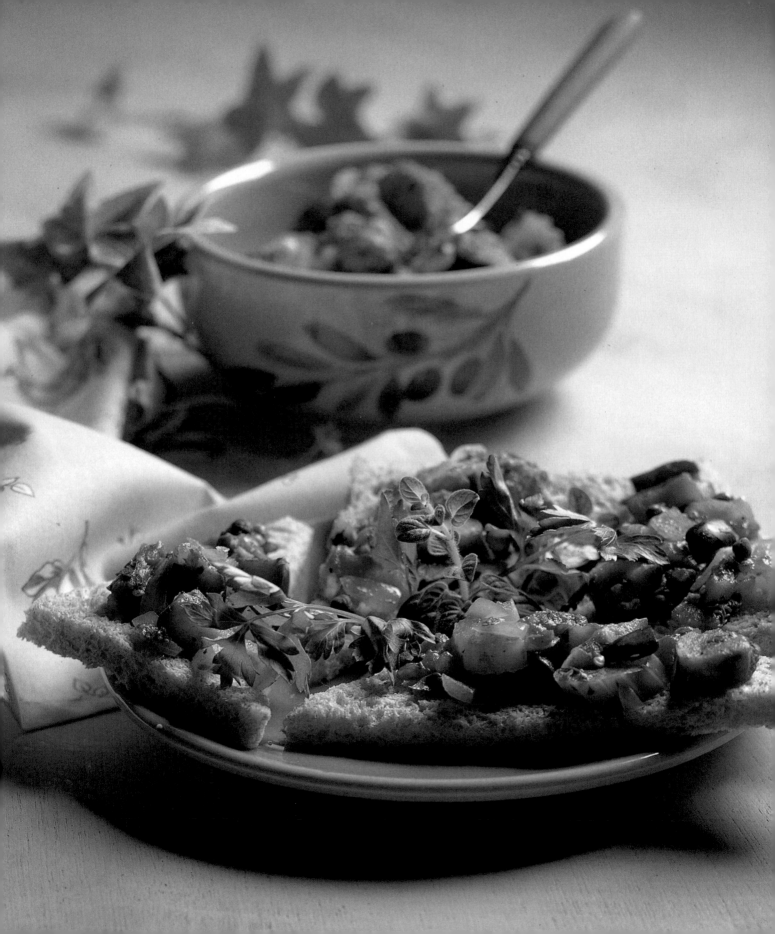

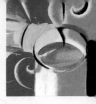

Caponata

Preparation: 20 minutes ✳ Cooking: 30 minutes ✳ Serves 12

Caponata is a traditional Italian appetizer, served as part of many anti-pasto arrays, and is made from a base of eggplant and tomatoes. Serve with the whole wheat bread, lowfat crackers or toasted pita wedges.

1 large globe eggplant (about 1 lb/
   500 g), peel intact, cut into
   1-inch (2.5-cm) cubes
2 teaspoons olive oil
1 onion, diced
2 garlic cloves, peeled and minced
2 celery stalks, chopped
2 tomatoes, chopped
¼ cup (2 fl oz/60 ml) red wine vinegar
6 large black olives, pitted and sliced
1½ tablespoons drained capers
2 tablespoons chopped fresh oregano
¼ teaspoon ground black pepper
2 tablespoons chopped fresh flat-leaf
   (Italian) parsley
24 slices whole wheat (wholemeal)
   bread

✳ Preheat an oven to 400°F (200°C). Coat a baking sheet with nonstick cooking spray.

✳ Spread the eggplant cubes on the baking sheet in a single layer. Bake for 15 minutes, turning halfway through the cooking time. Remove from the oven and set aside.

✳ In a large nonstick frying pan over medium heat, heat the oil. Add the onion, garlic and celery and sauté until tender, about 5 minutes.

✳ Add the baked eggplant, tomatoes, vinegar, olives, capers, oregano and pepper. Bring to a boil, reduce the heat to low and simmer until the caponata thickens, about 10 minutes. Remove from the heat and stir in the parsley.

✳ To serve, transfer to a serving bowl. Store in an airtight container in the refrigerator for up to 3 days. One serving is 2 slices of bread, each topped with 2 tablespoons of caponata.

Nutritional Analysis per Serving

Calories 172 (Kilojoules 723); Total fat 4g; Saturated fat 1g; Protein 6g; Cholesterol 0mg; Carbohydrates 32g; Sodium 355mg; Dietary fiber 5g; Calories from fat 17%

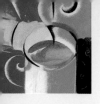

4⅓ cups (30 oz/940 g) cooked
     garbanzo beans, rinsed and drained
3 garlic cloves, peeled and minced
¼ cup (2 fl oz/60 ml) lemon juice
2 tablespoons tahini (sesame paste)
1 teaspoon ground cumin
1 teaspoon paprika
½ teaspoon finely grated lemon zest
½ teaspoon salt
4 pita breads, quartered

Hummus with Pita Bread

Preparation: 10 minutes ✳ *Serves 4*

✳ In a food processor with the metal blade or in a blender, combine the beans, garlic, lemon juice, tahini, cumin, paprika, lemon zest and salt. Process until smooth.

✳ To serve, use as a spread or dip with the pita bread. Makes 4 cups (28 oz/875 g). One serving is 2 tablespoons hummus and 1 pita bread. Store the hummus in an airtight container in the refrigerator for up to 3 days.

Nutritional Analysis per Serving

Calories 215 (Kilojoules 905); Total fat 2g; Saturated fat 0g; Protein 8g; Cholesterol 0mg; Carbohydrates 41g; Sodium 359mg; Dietary fiber 2g; Calories from fat 8%

2 teaspoons olive oil
2 small shallots, peeled and minced
1 garlic clove, minced
12 oz (375 g) fresh mushrooms, sliced
¼ cup (2 fl oz/60 ml) Chicken Stock
     (recipe on page 206) or reduced
     sodium chicken broth
2 tablespoons chopped fresh flat-leaf
     (Italian) parsley
1 tablespoon chopped fresh thyme
¼ teaspoon salt
¼ teaspoon ground black pepper
½ lb (250 g) sourdough bread, cut
     into eight 1-inch (2.5-cm) thick
     slices, toasted

Mushroom-Topped Crostini

Preparation: 15 minutes ✳ *Cooking: 15 minutes* ✳ *Serves 4*

✳ In a large nonstick frying pan over medium heat, heat the oil. Add the shallots and garlic and sauté until tender, about 2 minutes. Add the mushrooms and sauté for 5 minutes.

✳ Add the stock or broth, parsley, thyme, salt and pepper and simmer until the liquid evaporates, about 5 minutes. Remove from the heat and cool.

✳ Transfer the mixture to a food processor with the metal blade or to a blender and process into fine pieces.

✳ To serve, spread 2 tablespoons of the mushroom topping on each bread slice. One serving is 2 slices. Store the topping in an airtight container in the refrigerator for up to 3 days.

Nutritional Analysis per Serving

Calories 203 (Kilojoules 852); Total fat 4g; Saturated fat 1g; Protein 7g; Cholesterol 0mg; Carbohydrates 35g; Sodium 520mg; Dietary fiber 3g; Calories from fat 19%

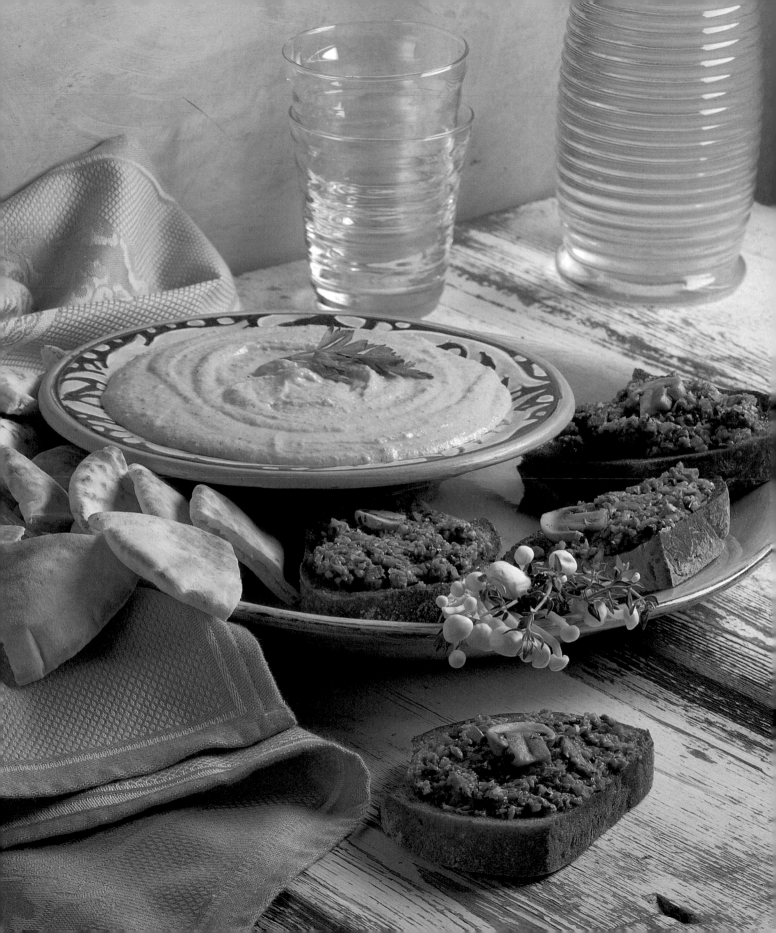

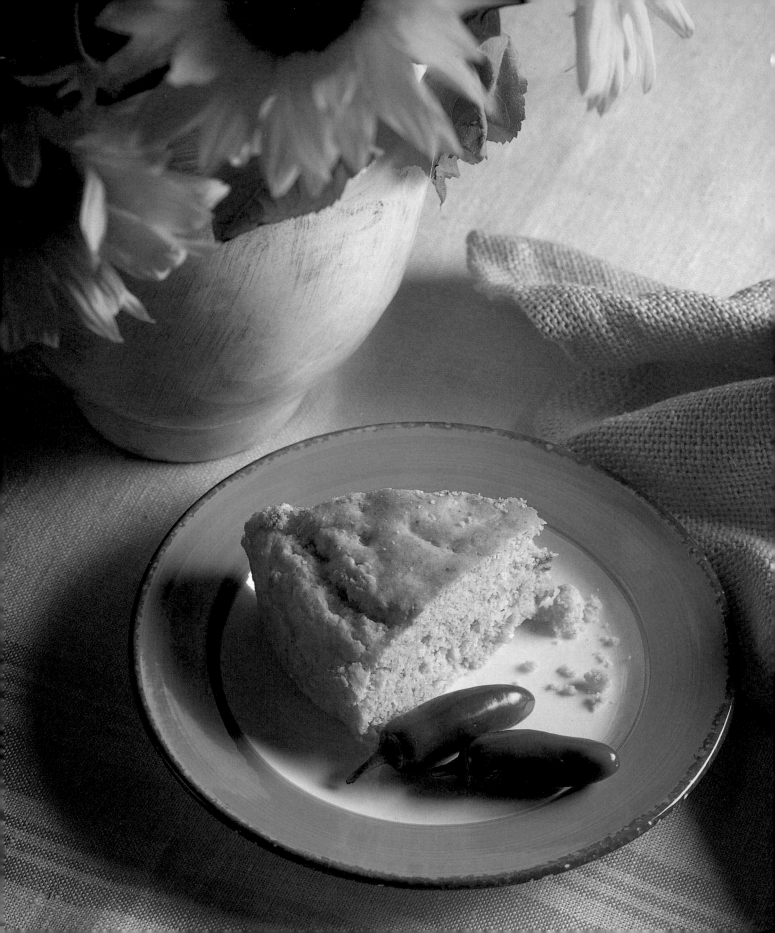

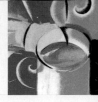

Chili-Cheese Corn Bread

Preparation: 20 minutes ✴ Cooking: 25 minutes ✴ Serves 8

This moist, flavorful bread makes a substantial side dish for soups and salads. The buttermilk used here replaces the sour cream in traditional Texan versions, greatly lowering the fat without lessening the taste.

✴ Preheat an oven to 400°F (200°C). Coat a 9-inch (23-cm) round cake pan with nonstick cooking spray.

✴ In a large bowl, combine the cornmeal, flour, baking powder, baking soda, salt and cayenne pepper. Make a well in the center.

✴ In a medium bowl, combine the egg whites, buttermilk, oil and honey and whisk until blended. Add the corn, cheese, chilies and pimientos and stir to mix well. Pour the egg mixture into the well in the dry ingredients and stir until just combined.

✴ Pour the batter into the prepared pan and bake until a toothpick inserted in the center comes out clean, about 20 minutes. Cool in the pan before slicing.

✴ To serve, cut into 8 pieces. One serving is 1 piece. Store wrapped in plastic wrap in the refrigerator for up to 3 days.

1 cup (5 oz/155 g) cornmeal

1 cup (5 oz/155 g) unbleached flour

2 teaspoons baking powder

½ teaspoon baking soda
   (bicarbonate of soda)

¾ teaspoon salt

¼ teaspoon cayenne pepper

2 egg whites

1 cup (8 fl oz/250 ml) lowfat
   buttermilk

2 tablespoons corn oil

2 tablespoons honey

1 cup (6 oz/185 g) corn kernels

⅓ cup (1½ oz/45 g) grated nonfat
   Monterey jack cheese

3 green chilies, seeded and chopped

1 tablespoon chopped pimientos
   (sweet peppers)

Shopping Tip

✴ Both green chilies and pimientos are available already seeded and chopped in cans and bottles, greatly lessening the preparation time of this bread.

Nutritional Analysis per Serving

Calories 226 (Kilojoules 951); Total fat 5g; Saturated fat 1g; Protein 8g; Cholesterol 1mg; Carbohydrates 39g; Sodium 499mg; Dietary fiber 2g; Calories from fat 18%

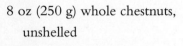

8 oz (250 g) whole chestnuts,
   unshelled

1 tablespoon olive oil

1 shallot, peeled and minced

1 garlic clove, peeled and minced

12 oz (375 g) spinach, stems trimmed

1 tablespoon balsamic vinegar

¼ teaspoon ground black pepper

Nutrition Tip

✳ Chestnuts are lower in fat than many counterparts in the nut family. Roasting brings out their flavor, while softening their texture. Toss chestnuts into your favorite salads, rice and pasta dishes for added protein and flavor.

1 lb (500 g) baby carrots

2 tablespoons chopped fresh dill

2 tablespoons orange juice

1 tablespoon olive oil

½ teaspoon finely grated lemon zest

¼ teaspoon ground mustard

¼ teaspoon salt

⅛ teaspoon ground black pepper

Spinach and Roasted Chestnuts

Preparation: 25 minutes ✳ *Cooking: 30 minutes* ✳ *Serves 4*

✳ Preheat an oven to 400°F (200°C).

✳ Using a sharp knife, cut an X in the flat side of each chestnut and spread the nuts in the bottom of a roasting pan. Roast until the shells split, 15–20 minutes. Cool to the touch. Remove and discard the shells and inner brown skin.

✳ In a large nonstick frying pan over medium heat, heat the oil. Add the shallot and garlic and sauté, stirring frequently, for 2 minutes. Add the spinach and vinegar and sauté, stirring frequently, until the spinach wilts, about 5 minutes. Add the pepper and chestnuts and sauté until the chestnuts are warm, about 5 minutes.

✳ To serve, divide among 4 individual plates.

Nutritional Analysis per Serving

Calories 136 (Kilojoules 570); Total fat 4g; Saturated fat 1g; Protein 3g; Cholesterol 0mg; Carbohydrates 23g; Sodium 50mg; Dietary fiber 2g; Calories from fat 27%

Steamed Carrots with Dill

Preparation: 15 minutes ✳ *Cooking: 10 minutes* ✳ *Serves 4*

✳ Fill a medium saucepan with 1 inch (2.5 cm) of water, set a steamer basket inside and place over medium heat. Add the carrots and steam until tender-crisp, 8–10 minutes.

✳ In a medium bowl, combine the dill, orange juice, olive oil, lemon zest, mustard, salt and pepper and whisk until blended.

✳ In a large bowl, combine the carrots and dill mixture and toss to mix well.

✳ To serve, divide among 4 individual plates.

Nutritional Analysis per Serving

Calories 84 (Kilojoules 353); Total fat 4g; Saturated fat 0g; Protein 1g; Cholesterol 0mg; Carbohydrates 13g; Sodium 176mg; Dietary fiber 4g; Calories from fat 37%

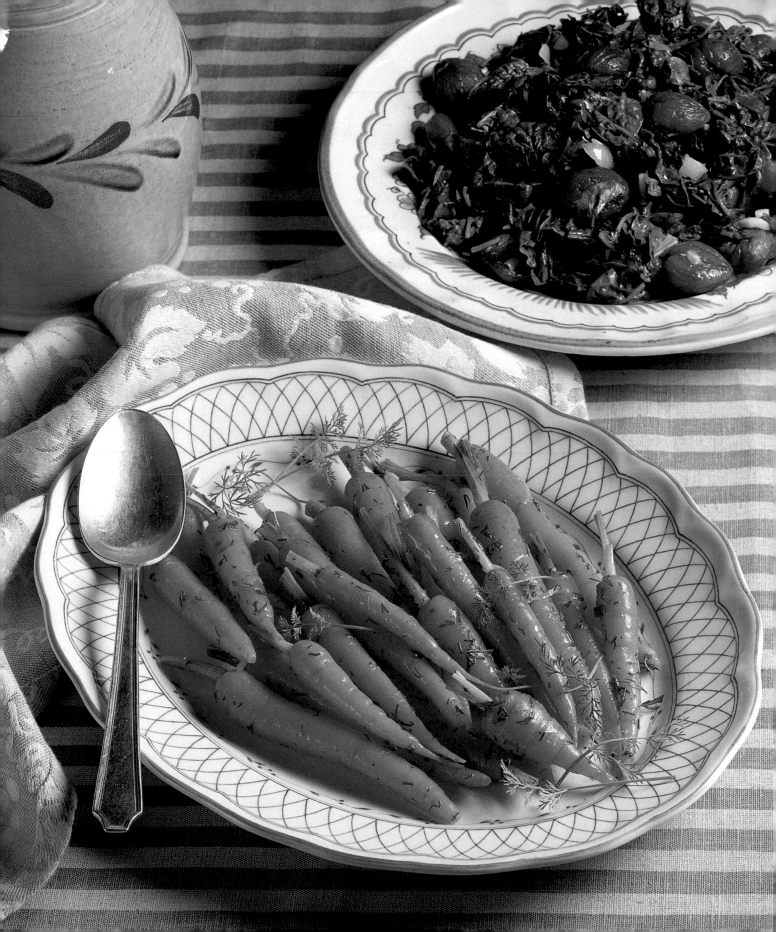

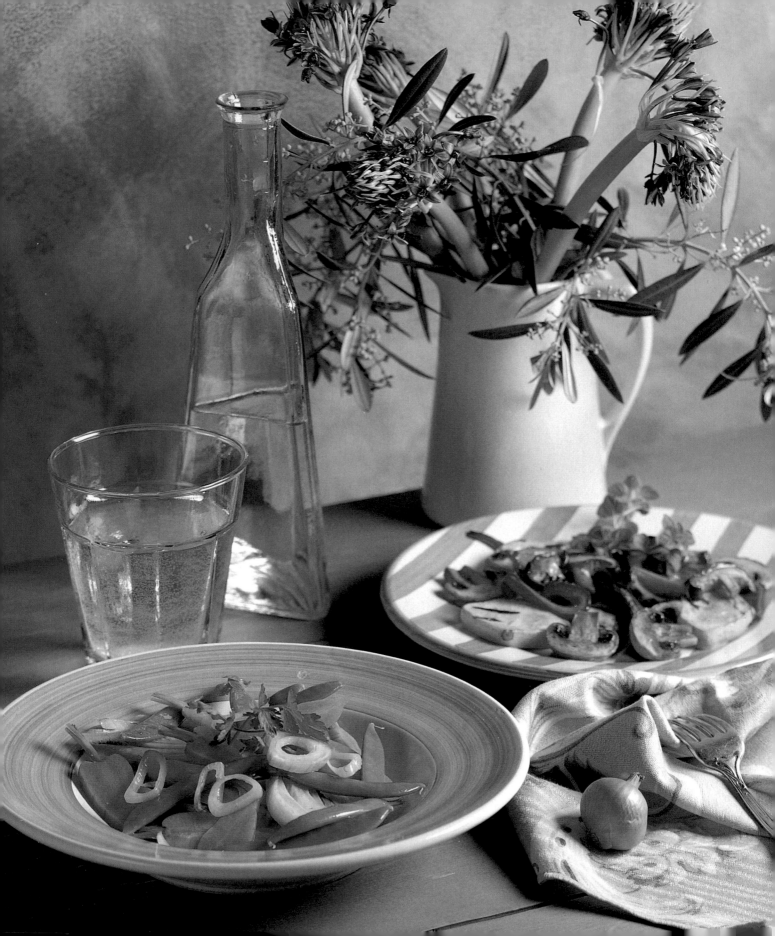

Grilled Summer Vegetables

2 tablespoons rice wine vinegar

1 tablespoon olive oil

1 tablespoon reduced sodium soy sauce

1 tablespoon Dijon-style mustard

1 tablespoon honey

1 red bell pepper (capsicum), seeded, deribbed and quartered

1 green bell pepper (capsicum), seeded, deribbed and quartered

1 green zucchini (courgette), halved lengthwise and crosswise

1 yellow zucchini (courgette), halved lengthwise and crosswise

10 large fresh mushrooms

Preparation: 30 minutes ✳ Cooking: 10 minutes ✳ Serves 4

✳ To make the marinade, in a large bowl, combine the vinegar, oil, soy sauce, mustard and honey and whisk until blended.

✳ Add the peppers, zucchini and mushrooms and toss to coat well. Cover, refrigerate and marinate for 15 minutes to 8 hours.

✳ Prepare a fire in an outdoor charcoal grill or preheat a broiler (griller). Place the vegetables on the grill or in the broiler and discard the marinade. Grill or broil for 5 minutes. Turn and grill or broil just until char marks appear, about 5 minutes more.

✳ To serve, divide among 4 individual plates.

Nutritional Analysis per Serving

Calories 94 (Kilojoules 396); Total fat 4g; Saturated fat 1g; Protein 3g; Cholesterol 0mg; Carbohydrates 13g; Sodium 247mg; Dietary fiber 2g; Calories from fat 34%

Spring Vegetable Sauté

1 teaspoon hazelnut (filbert) oil

8 oz (250 g) sugar snap peas

½ fennel bulb, peeled and thinly sliced

2 carrots, peeled and thinly sliced

2 shallots, peeled and thinly sliced

¼ teaspoon salt

Preparation: 10 minutes ✳ Cooking: 8 minutes ✳ Serves 4

All vegetable oils contain the antioxidant vitamin E, but hazelnut oil has the most. Even the scant amount used here—¼ teaspoon per serving—contains 4 percent of the recommended daily requirement.

✳ Coat a nonstick frying pan with nonstick cooking spray. Place over medium heat and heat the hazelnut oil. Add the peas, fennel, carrots, shallots and salt and sauté, stirring frequently, until tender-crisp, 5–8 minutes.

✳ To serve, divide among 4 individual plates.

Nutritional Analysis per Serving

Calories 68 (Kilojoules 286); Total fat 1g; Saturated fat 0g; Protein 3g; Cholesterol 0mg; Carbohydrates 12g; Sodium 246mg; Dietary fiber 3g; Calories from fat 19%

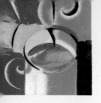

1 globe eggplant (aubergine), about
   1¼ lb (625 g), cut into 1-inch
   (2.5-cm) cubes

2 zucchini (courgettes), cut into 1-inch
   (2.5-cm) cubes

1 large onion, chopped

1 red bell pepper (capsicum), seeded,
   deribbed and cut into 1-inch
   (2.5-cm) cubes

1 green bell pepper (capsicum),
   seeded, deribbed and cut into
   1-inch (2.5-cm) cubes

2 garlic cloves, peeled and minced

2 tomatoes, chopped

1 tablespoon chopped fresh thyme

1 tablespoon fresh basil

¼ teaspoon salt

¼ teaspoon ground black pepper

Nutrition Tip

* Red bell peppers are especially high
in vitamin C, having more than twice as
much as green bell peppers—themselves
a good source of the vitamin.

Ratatouille

Preparation: 30 minutes * *Cooking: 35 minutes* * *Serves 4*

*This version of the traditional French stew features summer vegetables.
Substitute other seasonal produce and make the dish year-round.*

* Preheat a broiler (griller). Coat a large baking sheet with nonstick cooking spray. Spread the eggplant cubes on the prepared
sheet and lightly coat with cooking spray.

* Broil (grill) until golden, about 7 minutes, turning halfway
through the cooking time. Remove the baking sheet from the
oven, add the zucchini, onion and bell peppers and lightly coat
with nonstick cooking spray.

* Broil (grill) until browned, turning halfway through the
cooking time, about 8 minutes more.

* Coat a large nonstick frying pan with nonstick cooking
spray and place over medium heat. Add the garlic and sauté for
2 minutes.

* Add the tomatoes, thyme, basil, salt and pepper, reduce the
heat to low and simmer for 5 minutes.

* Add the vegetables to the tomato mixture and stir to mix
well. Cover and simmer until the liquid is reduced by half, about
10 minutes.

* To serve, divide among 4 individual plates.

Nutritional Analysis per Serving

Calories 102 (Kilojoules 430); Total fat 1g; Saturated fat 0g; Protein 4g;
Cholesterol 0mg; Carbohydrates 22g; Sodium 152mg; Dietary fiber 5g;
Calories from fat 10%

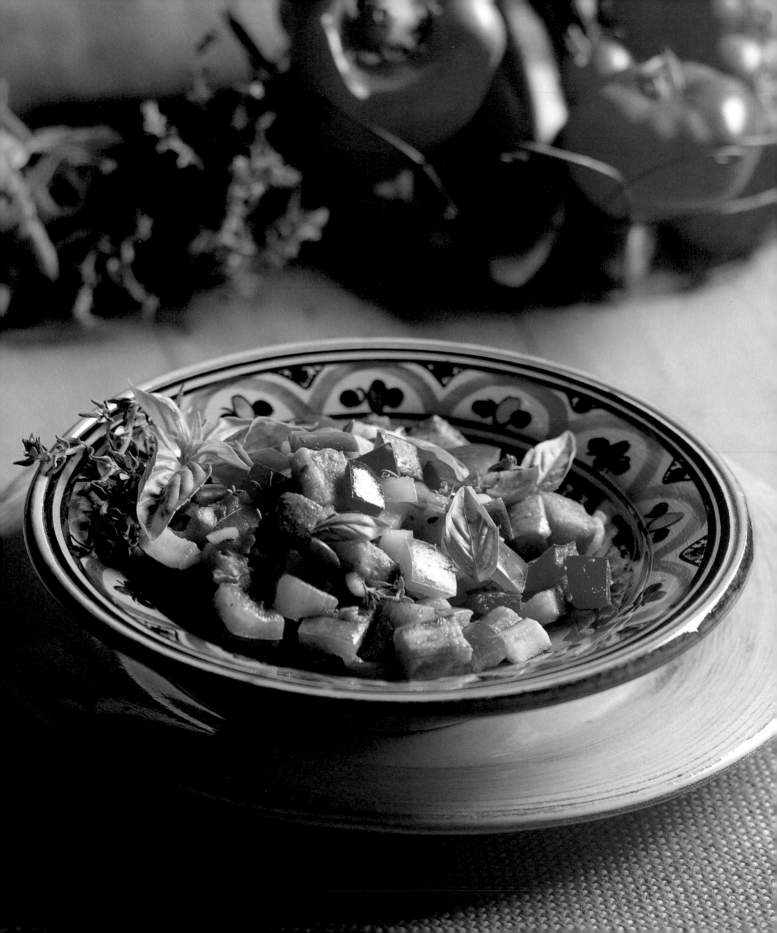

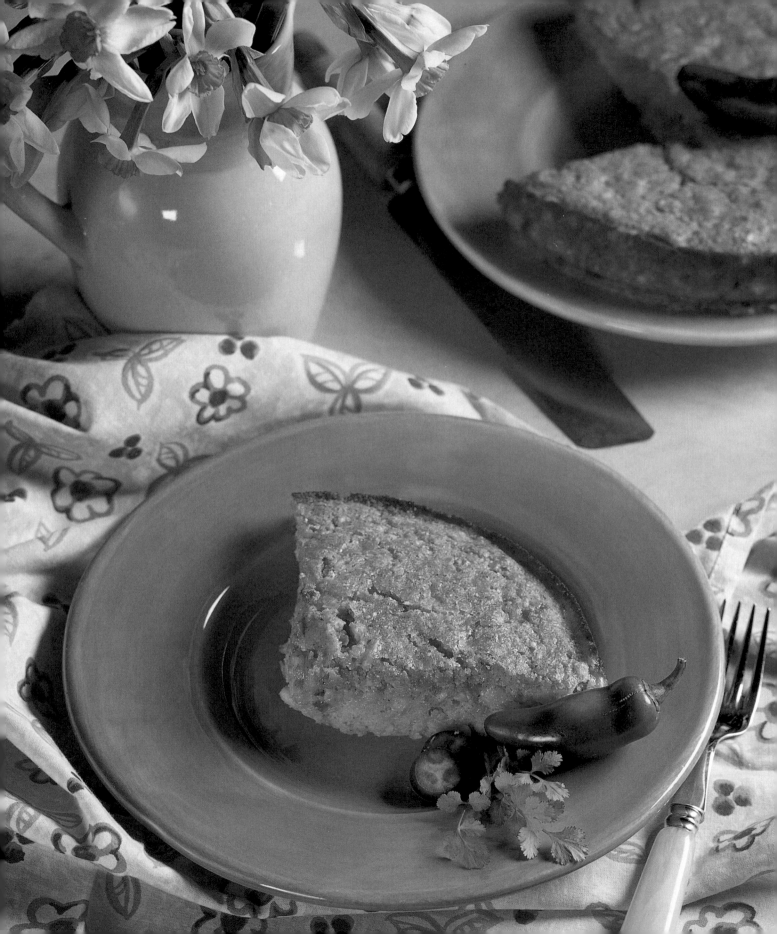

Corn Pudding

1 cup (5 oz/155 g) stone-ground
    yellow cornmeal (maize flour)

2 teaspoons baking powder

1 teaspoon chili powder

½ teaspoon salt

2 cups (12 oz/375 g) corn kernels

3 tablespoons honey

1 cup (8 fl oz/250 ml) lowfat
    buttermilk

3 tablespoons safflower oil

3 egg whites

½ cup (2 oz/60 g) grated reduced fat
    Monterey jack cheese

3 green chilies, seeded and chopped

Storage Tip

✳ Store this side dish wrapped in plastic
in the refrigerator for up to 2 days.

Preparation: 20 minutes ✳ *Cooking: 40 minutes* ✳ *Serves 4*

*This recipe makes four generous servings of this hearty side dish. Use it
as an alternative to bread or rolls. Each serving fulfills both a grain and
a vegetable requirement of a healthy daily diet.*

✳ Preheat an oven to 350°F (180°C). Coat a 9-inch (23-cm)
round cake pan with nonstick cooking spray.

✳ In a large bowl, combine the cornmeal, baking powder, chili
powder and salt. Make a well in the center.

✳ In another large bowl, using a wire whisk, combine the corn,
honey, buttermilk, oil and egg whites. Add the cheese and chilies
and stir to mix well.

✳ Pour the corn mixture into the well in the dry ingredients
and stir until blended. Transfer to the prepared pan and bake until
golden and a toothpick inserted in the center comes out clean,
about 30 minutes. Cool in the pan for 10 minutes before slicing.

✳ To serve, divide among 4 individual plates.

Nutritional Analysis per Serving

Calories 437 (Kilojoules 1,835); Total fat 15g; Saturated fat 3g; Protein 16g;
Cholesterol 12mg; Carbohydrates 64g; Sodium 756mg; Dietary fiber 5g;
Calories from fat 30%

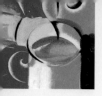

3 large baking potatoes, about 1½ lb
   (750 g), peeled

4 cups (32 fl oz/1 l) water

1 tablespoon white wine vinegar

2 egg whites

1 teaspoon paprika

½ teaspoon salt

Baked French Fries

Preparation: 35 minutes ✳ *Cooking: 40 minutes* ✳ *Serves 4*

✳ Slice the potatoes lengthwise into matchsticks, about ¼ inch (6 mm) thick. In a large bowl, combine the water, vinegar and potatoes. Set aside, uncovered, for 15 minutes at room temperature.

✳ In a small bowl, using an electric mixer on high speed, beat the egg whites until foamy.

✳ Preheat an oven to 400°F (200°C). Coat a large baking sheet with nonstick cooking spray.

✳ Place the potatoes on the prepared baking sheet in a single layer. Brush the tops and sides with the beaten egg whites and sprinkle with the paprika and salt. Bake, turning several times, until golden brown and crisp, about 40 minutes.

✳ To serve, divide among 4 individual plates.

Nutritional Analysis per Serving

Calories 138 (Kilojoules 579); Total fat 1g; Saturated fat 0g; Protein 6g; Cholesterol 0mg; Carbohydrates 29g; Sodium 313mg; Dietary fiber 3g; Calories from fat 3%

3 large baking potatoes, about 1½ lb
   (750 g), peeled and cut into
   2-inch (5-cm) chunks

2 tablespoons chopped fresh rosemary

½ teaspoon ground black pepper

Rosemary Roasted Potatoes

Preparation: 10 minutes ✳ *Cooking: 1 hour* ✳ *Serves 4*

✳ Preheat an oven to 400°F (200°C). On a large baking sheet, spread out the potatoes and lightly coat the tops and sides with nonstick cooking spray. Sprinkle with the rosemary and pepper.

✳ Bake, turning every 15 minutes, until golden brown and tender in the middle, about 1 hour.

✳ To serve, divide among 4 individual plates.

Nutritional Analysis per Serving

Calories 135 (Kilojoules 565); Total fat 1g; Saturated fat 0g; Protein 4g; Cholesterol 0mg; Carbohydrates 29g; Sodium 12mg; Dietary fiber 3g; Calories from fat 8%

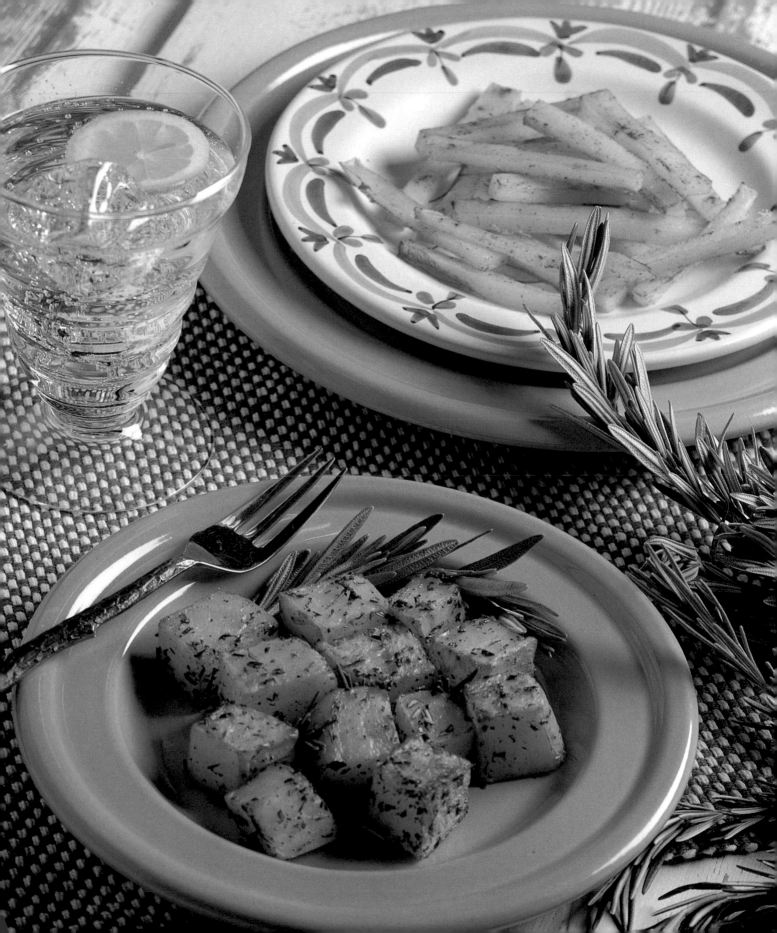

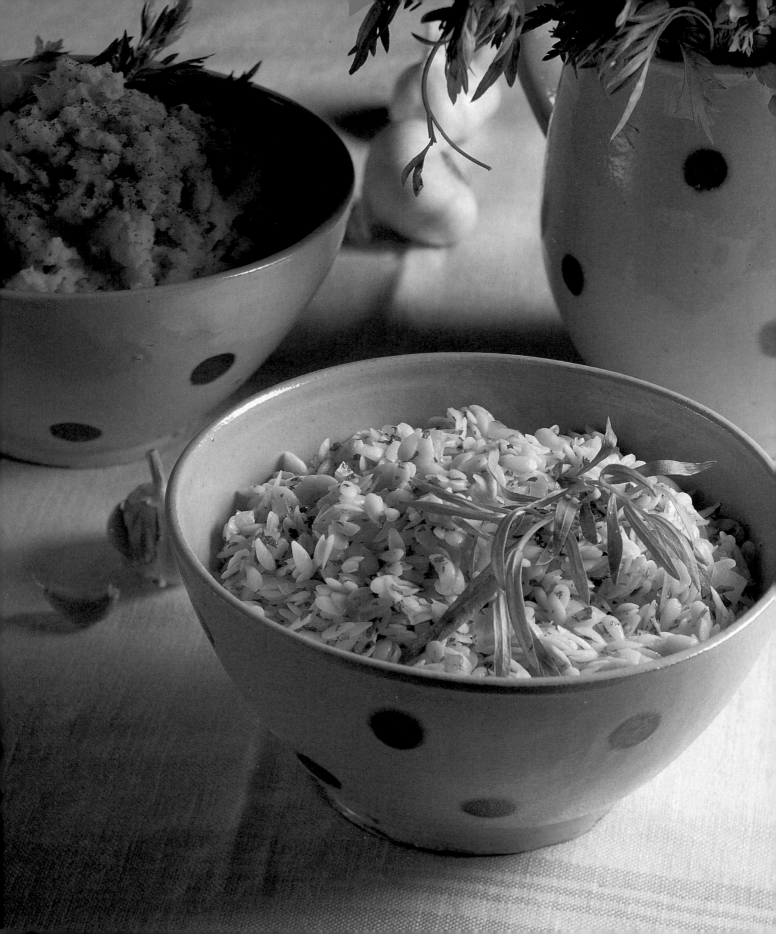

Garlic Mashed Potatoes

4 large baking potatoes, about 2 lb
(1 kg), scrubbed and quartered

4 garlic cloves, peeled

6 cups (48 fl oz/1.5 l) water

½ cup (4 fl oz/125 ml) lowfat
buttermilk

½ teaspoon ground black pepper

¼ teaspoon ground nutmeg

¼ cup (⅓ oz/10 g) chopped fresh
flat-leaf (Italian) parsley

*Preparation: 15 minutes * Cooking: 15 minutes * Serves 4*

✳ In a large saucepan over high heat, combine the potatoes, garlic and water. Bring to a boil, reduce the heat to low, cover and simmer until the potatoes are tender when pierced with a fork, about 15 minutes. Drain, reserving ¼ cup (2 fl oz/60 ml) of the cooking water.

✳ In a large bowl, combine the potatoes and garlic, reserved cooking water, buttermilk, pepper and nutmeg. Using an electric mixer on high speed or a potato masher, mash until smooth, about 2 minutes by machine or 5 minutes by hand. Add the parsley and stir to mix well.

✳ To serve, divide among 4 individual plates.

Nutritional Analysis per Serving

Calories 199 (Kilojoules 835); Total fat 1g; Saturated fat 0g; Protein 6g; Cholesterol 2mg; Carbohydrates 43g; Sodium 59mg; Dietary fiber 4g; Calories from fat 3%

Nutrition Tip

✳ Substituting lowfat buttermilk for the traditional whole milk and butter gives these mashed potatoes plenty of taste but far fewer fat grams and calories. Leaving the skins intact increases the vitamins and fiber and provides an appealing texture.

Orzo with Shallots and Herbs

8 cups (64 fl oz/2 l) water

8 oz (250 g) dried orzo

3 shallots, peeled and chopped

½ cup (4 fl oz/125 ml) Chicken Stock
(recipe on page 206) or reduced
sodium chicken broth

1 tablespoon chopped fresh basil

1 tablespoon chopped fresh oregano

1 tablespoon chopped fresh tarragon

¼ teaspoon salt

¼ teaspoon ground black pepper

*Preparation: 20 minutes * Cooking: 10 minutes * Serves 4*

✳ In a large saucepan over high heat, bring the water to a boil. Add the orzo and shallots and cook until the orzo is tender, about 10 minutes. Drain.

✳ In a large bowl, combine the stock or broth, basil, oregano, tarragon, salt and pepper. Add the orzo and shallots and stir to mix well.

✳ To serve, divide among 4 individual plates. Serve hot or cold.

Nutritional Analysis per Serving

Calories 220 (Kilojoules 926); Total fat 1g; Saturated fat 0g; Protein 8g; Cholesterol 0mg; Carbohydrates 44g; Sodium 210mg; Dietary fiber 1g; Calories from fat 4%

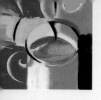

3 lb (1.5 kg) chicken pieces, including
   necks and backs if desired

3 onions, chopped

4 carrots, peeled and chopped

4 celery stalks with leaves, chopped

2 fresh flat-leaf (Italian) parsley sprigs

5 fresh thyme sprigs

2 bay leaves

1 teaspoon salt

8 whole black peppercorns

3 qt (3 l) water

Cooking Tip

✳ Substitute a whole roast bird from
which you have eaten half the meat for
the chicken pieces, if desired.

Chicken Stock

Preparation: 15 minutes ✳ Cooking: 2 hours 40 minutes ✳ Makes 3 qt (3 l)

*Homemade chicken stock is indispensable as a foundation for soups, stews
and chowders. When you make your own, you can season the stock with
your favorite herbs and spices and add the amount of sodium that best
suits your dietary needs. This is the kind of cooking you can do while
busy with other tasks around the house.*

✳ In a large stockpot over high heat, combine the chicken pieces,
onions, carrots, celery, parsley, thyme, bay leaves, salt, peppercorns
and water, increase the heat to high and bring to a boil. Reduce
the heat to medium-high and boil, uncovered, for 15 minutes.
Using paper towels, skim the foam that rises to the surface. Reduce
the heat to low, cover and simmer for 2 hours, skimming the
surface as needed. Remove from the heat and cool 20 minutes.

✳ Strain the stock through a fine-mesh sieve over a large bowl to
remove the solids, pressing hard on the chicken and vegetables to
extract their full flavor. Cover and refrigerate for at least 8 hours.

✳ Using paper towels, skim the congealed fat from the cold
stock. Transfer to airtight containers and refrigerate for up to
3 days or freeze for up to 3 months. For nutritional analysis, one
serving is 1 cup (8 fl oz/250 ml).

Nutritional Analysis per Serving

Calories 27 (Kilojoules 114); Total fat 2g; Saturated fat 1g; Protein 3g;
Cholesterol 0mg; Carbohydrates 2g; Sodium 300mg; Dietary fiber 0g;
Calories from fat 50%

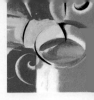

Vegetable Stock

Preparation: 20 minutes ✳ *Cooking: 1 hour* ✳ *Makes 4 qt (4 l)*

This vegetable stock is a wonderful nonfat base for soups, stews and sauces. Also, use it whenever water is called for in rice and whole-grain dishes to add flavor and nutrients.

5 carrots, peeled and chopped

5 celery stalks, with leaves, chopped

2 onions, quartered

½ cup (½ oz/15 g) chopped fresh
    flat-leaf (Italian) parsley

5 fresh thyme sprigs

2 fresh oregano sprigs

10 whole black peppercorns

1 dried red chili pepper, halved

4 qt (4 l) water

✳ In a large stockpot over high heat, combine the carrots, celery, onions, parsley, thyme, oregano, peppercorns, chili pepper and water. Bring to a boil, reduce the heat to medium and simmer, covered, for 1 hour. Remove from the heat and cool 20 minutes.

✳ Strain the stock through a fine-mesh sieve over a large bowl to remove the solids, pressing hard on the vegetables to extract their full flavor. Transfer to airtight containers and refrigerate for up to 3 days or freeze for up to 3 months. For nutritional analysis, one serving is 1 cup (8 fl oz/250 ml).

Storage Tip

✳ Make the stock ahead and store in airtight containers such as sealable plastic freezer bags or bottles. For convenience, freeze the stock in ice-cube trays and use the frozen cubes as necessary. The stock keeps in the refrigerator for up to 3 days or in the freezer for up to 3 months.

Nutritional Analysis per Serving

Calories 13 (Kilojoules 56); Total fat 0g; Saturated fat 0g; Protein 0g; Cholesterol 0mg; Carbohydrates 3g; Sodium 16mg; Dietary fiber 1g; Calories from fat 3%

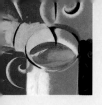

2 teaspoons olive oil

1 garlic clove, peeled and minced

2 teaspoons grated fresh ginger

⅛ teaspoon crushed red pepper flakes

1 cup (7 oz/220 g) uncooked
   basmati rice

¼ cup sliced (flaked) almonds

1 bay leaf

2 cups (16 fl oz/500 ml) Chicken
   Stock (recipe on page 206) or
   reduced sodium chicken broth

½ teaspoon salt

2 teaspoons vegetable oil

2 garlic cloves, peeled and minced

1 celery stalk, chopped

¾ cup (4½ oz/140 g) uncooked
   wild rice

½ cup (3 oz/90 g) chopped mixed
   dried fruit (prunes, pears, apples
   and apricots)

2½ cups (20 fl oz/625 ml) Chicken
   Stock (recipe on page 206) or
   reduced sodium chicken broth

2 tablespoons chopped fresh thyme

1 tablespoon chopped fresh sage

¼ teaspoon ground black pepper

Spicy Rice Pilaf

Preparation: 15 minutes ✳ *Cooking: 25 minutes* ✳ *Serves 4*

✳ In a medium saucepan over medium heat, heat the oil. Add the garlic, ginger and red pepper flakes and sauté, stirring frequently, for 2 minutes. Add the rice, almonds and bay leaf and sauté, stirring frequently, until the rice is golden, about 3 minutes more. Add the stock or broth and salt, increase the heat to medium-high and bring to a boil.

✳ Reduce the heat to low, cover and simmer until the liquid is absorbed, about 20 minutes.

✳ To serve, remove and discard the bay leaf, fluff with a fork and divide among 4 individual plates.

Nutritional Analysis per Serving

Calories 234 (Kilojoules 983); Total fat 6g; Saturated fat 1g; Protein 7g; Cholesterol 0mg; Carbohydrates 40g; Sodium 576mg; Dietary fiber 1g; Calories from fat 23%

Wild Rice with Mixed Dried Fruit

Preparation: 20 minutes ✳ *Cooking: 1 hour 10 minutes* ✳ *Serves 4*

✳ In a medium saucepan over medium heat, heat the oil. Add the garlic and celery and sauté for 2 minutes. Add the rice and mixed dried fruit and sauté for 2 minutes more.

✳ Add the stock or broth, thyme, sage and pepper, increase the heat to medium-high and bring to a boil.

✳ Reduce the heat to low, cover and simmer, stirring occasionally, for 1 hour. Uncover and simmer until the liquid is absorbed, about 5 minutes more.

✳ To serve, fluff with a fork and divide among 4 individual plates.

Nutritional Analysis per Serving

Calories 204 (Kilojoules 857); Total fat 3g; Saturated fat 0g; Protein 7g; Cholesterol 0mg; Carbohydrates 39g; Sodium 365mg; Dietary fiber 3g; Calories from fat 12%

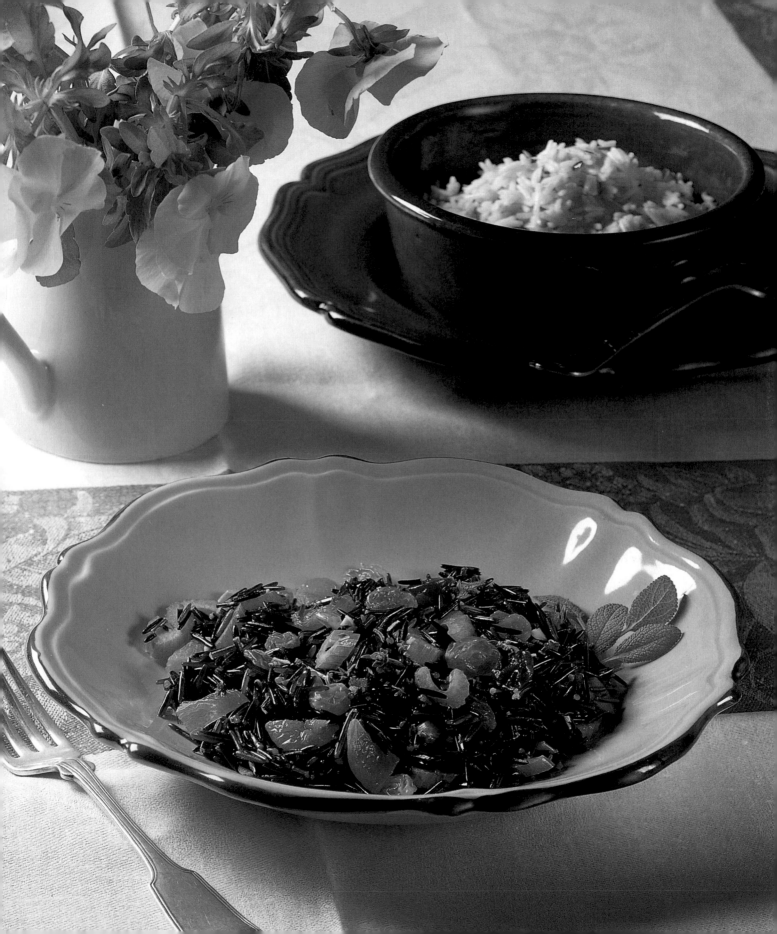

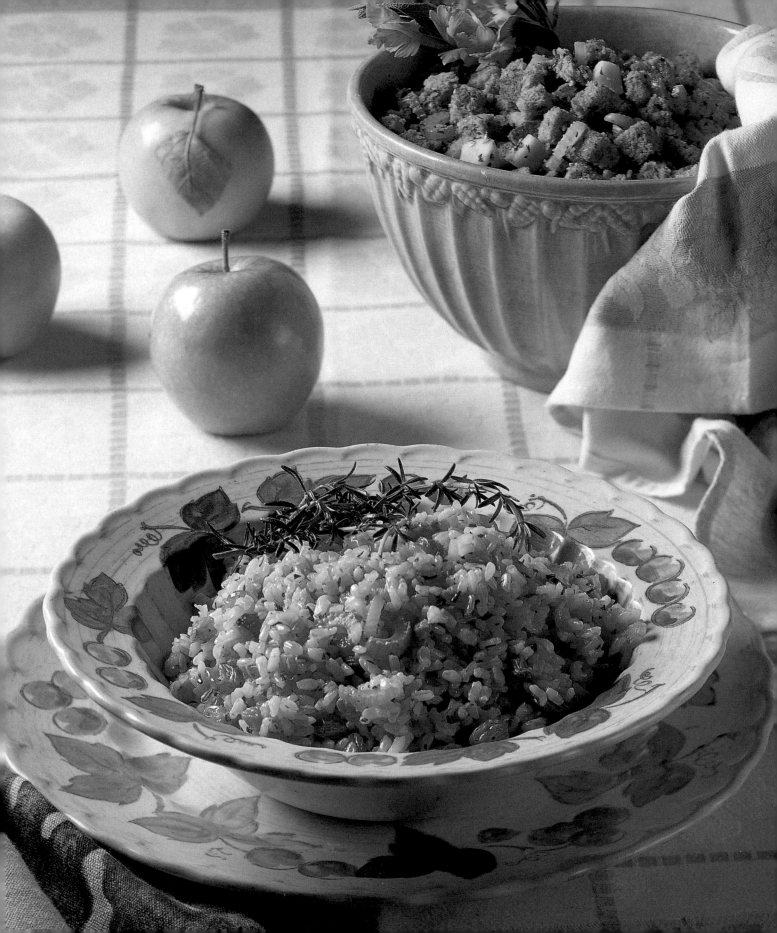

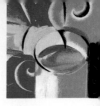

1 tablespoon margarine

1 large onion, chopped

4 celery stalks, chopped

1 tart apple, such as Granny Smith, peeled, cored and cubed

¼ cup (⅓ oz/10 g) chopped fresh flat-leaf (Italian) parsley

2 tablespoons chopped fresh oregano

2 teaspoons chopped fresh sage

1 tablespoon chopped fresh rosemary

¼ teaspoon ground black pepper

5 cups (10 oz/315 g) whole wheat (wholemeal) bread cubes, lightly toasted

2 cups (16 fl oz/500 ml) Chicken Stock (recipe on page 206) or reduced sodium chicken broth

Bread and Apple Dressing

Preparation: 25 minutes ✳ Cooking: 30 minutes ✳ Serves 4

✳ Preheat an oven to 350°F (180°C). Coat a 2-qt (2-l) baking dish with nonstick cooking spray.

✳ In a large nonstick frying pan over medium heat, melt the margarine. Add the onion, celery and apple and sauté, stirring frequently, for 5 minutes. Add the parsley, oregano, sage, rosemary and pepper and stir to mix well.

✳ Transfer the mixture to a large bowl and add the bread cubes and stock or broth. Toss to mix well. Pour into the prepared dish and bake, uncovered, until golden brown and the liquid is absorbed, about 25 minutes. To serve, divide among 4 individual plates.

Nutritional Analysis per Serving

Calories 262 (Kilojoules 1,100); Total fat 6g; Saturated fat 1g; Protein 9g; Cholesterol 0mg; Carbohydrates 45g; Sodium 72mg; Dietary fiber 7g; Calories from fat 21%

2 teaspoons olive oil

2 shallots, peeled and minced

2 celery stalks, diced

1 cup (7 oz/220 g) uncooked brown rice

2¼ cups (18 fl oz/560 ml) Chicken Stock (recipe on page 206) or reduced sodium chicken broth

½ cup (3 oz/90 g) golden raisins (sultanas)

2 tablespoons chopped fresh rosemary

¼ teaspoon salt

¼ teaspoon ground black pepper

Rice, Raisin and Rosemary Dressing

Preparation: 20 minutes ✳ Cooking: 1 hour ✳ Serves 4

✳ Preheat an oven to 350°F (180°C). Coat a 2-qt (2-l) baking dish with nonstick cooking spray.

✳ In a medium saucepan over medium heat, heat the oil. Add the shallots and celery and sauté, stirring frequently, for 3 minutes. Add the rice and sauté until golden, about 3 minutes more. Add the stock or broth, raisins, rosemary, salt and pepper and bring to a boil. Reduce the heat to low, cover and simmer for 15 minutes.

✳ Transfer to the prepared dish and bake, uncovered, until golden, about 40 minutes. To serve, divide among 4 individual plates.

Nutritional Analysis per Serving

Calories 289 (Kilojoules 1,213); Total fat 4g; Saturated fat 1g; Protein 6g; Cholesterol 0mg; Carbohydrates 57g; Sodium 474mg; Dietary fiber 3g; Calories from fat 13%

3½ cups (28 fl oz/875 ml) water

2 tablespoons lemon juice

4 large tart apples such as
  Granny Smith

½ cup (2 oz/60 g) dried cranberries

3 tablespoons sugar

1 cinnamon stick, about 3 inches
  (7.5 cm) long

1 teaspoon finely grated lemon zest

Storage Tip

✳ To chill the dessert, cool at room temperature for 20 minutes. Transfer to an airtight container and refrigerate for up to 4 days. For the best results, allow the compote to sit at room temperature for 15 minutes before serving.

Cranberry-Applesauce

Preparation: 15 minutes ✳ Cooking: 15 minutes ✳ Serves 4

This dessert is delicious served hot or cold paired with grilled chicken, pork and game dishes. It makes a great breakfast side dish, too.

✳ In a medium bowl, combine 2 cups (16 fl oz/500 ml) of the water and 1 tablespoon of the lemon juice.

✳ Peel and core the apples and slice into 1-inch (2.5-cm) chunks, dropping the chunks into the water and lemon mixture to prevent browning.

✳ In a medium saucepan over medium-high heat, combine the remaining water and lemon juice and the cranberries, sugar and cinnamon stick and bring to a boil.

✳ Drain the apples, discard the water and add the apples to the saucepan. Reduce the heat to low and simmer, partially covered, until the apples are tender when pierced with a fork but still whole, about 5 minutes. Using a slotted spoon, transfer the apples and cranberries to a serving bowl.

✳ Increase the heat to high and bring the remaining liquid and cinnamon stick to a boil. Boil until the liquid is reduced by a third. Remove from the heat, remove and discard the cinnamon stick and stir in the lemon zest.

✳ Pour the syrup over the apples and cranberries and stir, mashing slightly.

✳ To serve, divide among 4 individual bowls.

Nutritional Analysis per Serving

Calories 167 (Kilojoules 700); Total fat 1g; Saturated fat 0g; Protein 0g; Cholesterol 0mg; Carbohydrates 43g; Sodium 1mg; Dietary fiber 4g; Calories from fat 3%

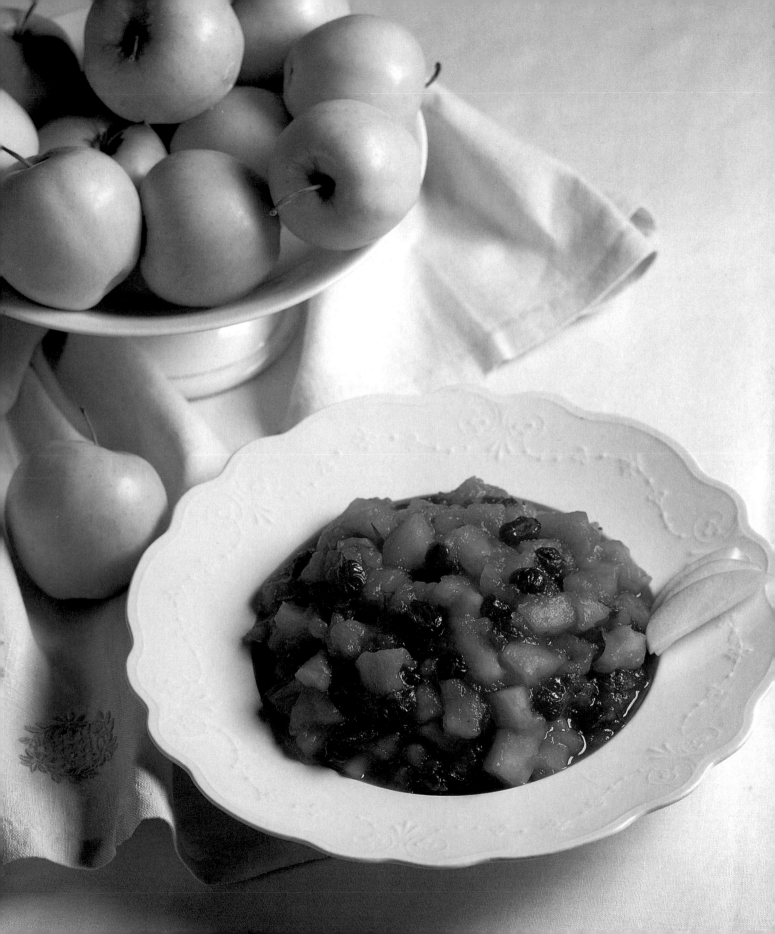

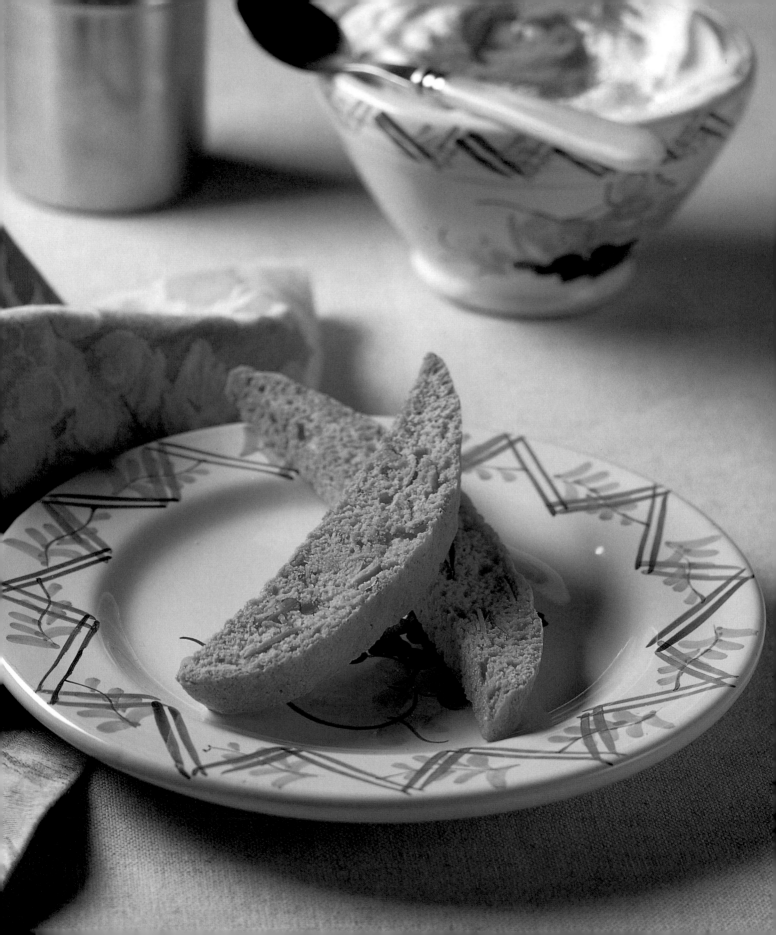

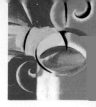

2 cups (10 oz/315 g) unbleached flour

1 cup (8 oz/250 g) sugar

½ cup (2 oz/60 g) sliced (flaked)
  almonds, toasted

¾ teaspoon baking soda
  (bicarbonate of soda)

¼ teaspoon salt

2 eggs

2 egg whites

1 teaspoon vanilla extract (essence)

½ teaspoon almond extract (essence)

Cooking Tip

✻ To toast almonds, or any kind of shelled nut, spread on a baking sheet and toast in a 350°F (180°C) oven until lightly golden, 4–5 minutes, tossing the nuts halfway through the cooking time.

Almond Biscotti

Preparation: 20 minutes ✻ Cooking: 55 minutes ✻ Serves 18

These crisp Italian cookies—the name means "twice baked"—are wonderful for dipping into a hot drink. Serve them as a lowfat dessert, breakfast pastry or lowfat snack. They're an excellent choice for making ahead and having on hand for unexpected guests as they will keep in an airtight container for up to 1 week. The taste actually improves after a day or two of storage.

✻ Preheat an oven to 325°F (165°C). Coat a baking sheet with nonstick cooking spray.

✻ In a large bowl, combine the flour, sugar, almonds, baking soda and salt. In a medium bowl, whisk together the eggs, egg whites, and vanilla and almond extracts. Add the egg mixture to the dry ingredients and stir until just blended. Turn the dough onto a well-floured work surface and shape into a smooth ball. Shape into a 10-inch-long (25-cm) log and place on the prepared baking sheet. Bake until a toothpick inserted in the center comes out clean, 30–35 minutes. Cool for 5 minutes.

✻ Reduce the oven to 300°F (150°C). Place the log on a work surface and slice into 18 pieces. Arrange the slices on the baking sheet and bake, turning once about halfway through, until golden brown, about 20 minutes. Cool until crisp.

✻ Store in an airtight container at room temperature for up to 1 week. One serving is 1 cookie.

Nutritional Analysis per Serving

Calories 136 (Kilojoules 573); Total fat 2g; Saturated fat 0g; Protein 3g; Cholesterol 24mg; Carbohydrates 25g; Sodium 96mg; Dietary fiber 1g; Calories from fat 16%

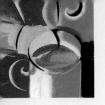

2 cups (10 oz/315 g) unbleached flour

1 cup (3 oz/90 g) rolled oats

¾ cup (3 oz/90 g) chopped pecans, lightly toasted

1 teaspoon baking soda (bicarbonate of soda)

¼ teaspoon salt

8 oz (250 g) nonfat cream cheese

2 tablespoons margarine

½ cup (4 oz/125 g) sugar

½ cup (4 fl oz/125 ml) orange juice

2 tablespoons nonfat vanilla yogurt

1 egg

1 egg white

1 tablespoon finely grated orange zest

1 teaspoon vanilla extract (essence)

1½ cups (6 oz/185 g) confectioners' (icing) sugar

Orange-Pecan Drop Cookies

Preparation: 20 minutes ✳ *Cooking: 15 minutes* ✳ *Serves 20*

A refreshing orange flavor permeates this twist on oatmeal drop cookies. I recommend you add these to your baking repertoire. While they are sweet enough to satisfy even my sugar cravings, the use of orange juice, nonfat cream cheese and yogurt, rather than lots of sugar and butter, keeps them relatively low calorie and lowfat.

✳ Preheat an oven to 350°F (180°C). Coat 2 large baking sheets with nonstick cooking spray.

✳ In a medium bowl, combine the flour, oats, pecans, baking soda and salt. In a food processor with the metal blade or in a large bowl, combine the cream cheese, margarine and sugar. Process or stir until smooth. Add half of the orange juice, the yogurt, egg, egg white, orange zest and vanilla. Process or stir until smooth. Gradually add the flour mixture and process or stir until just blended.

✳ Drop about 60 rounded tablespoons onto the prepared baking sheets. Bake until golden at the edges, about 15 minutes.

✳ To make the glaze, in a small bowl, combine the remaining orange juice and the confectioners' sugar and whisk until smooth. Using a pastry brush, coat the warm cookies with the glaze.

✳ Store in an airtight container at room temperature for up to 1 week. One serving is 3 cookies.

Nutritional Analysis per Serving

Calories 182 (Kilojoules 764); Total fat 5g; Saturated fat 1g; Protein 5g; Cholesterol 12mg; Carbohydrates 30g; Sodium 165mg; Dietary fiber 1g; Calories from fat 23%

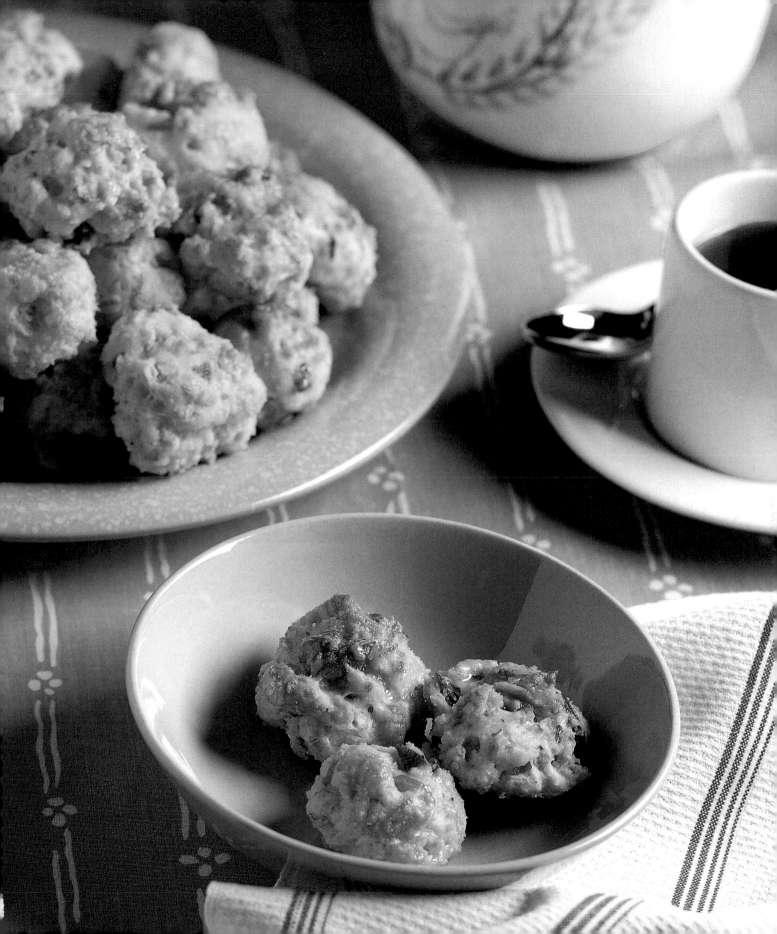

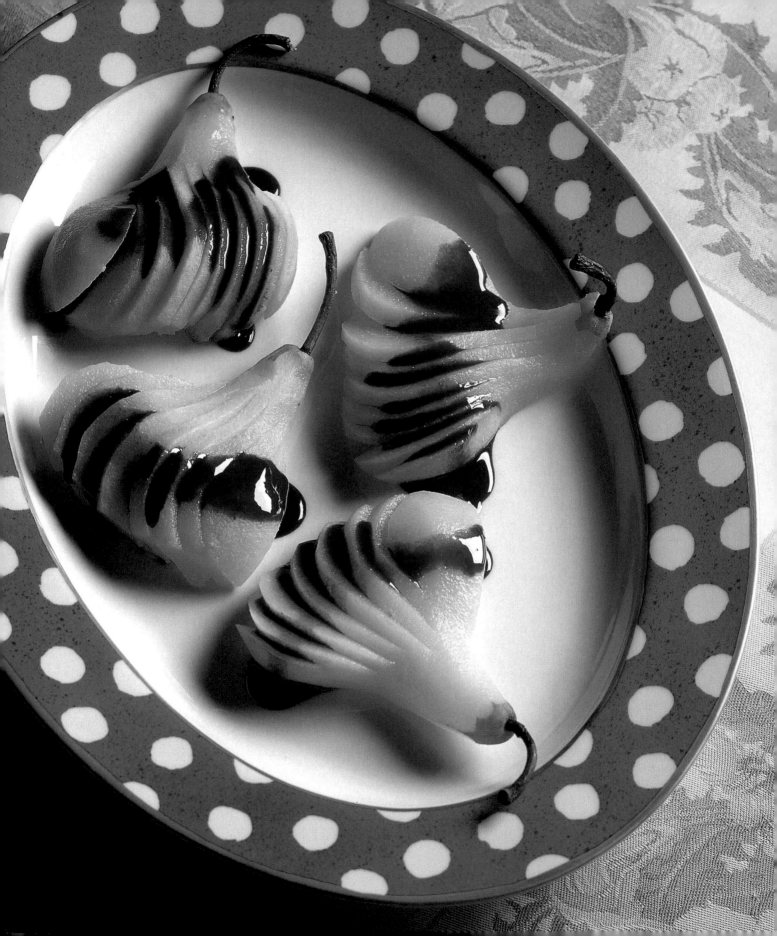

Pears with Chocolate Sauce

4 firm Anjou or Bosc pears, peeled,
  halved and cored

2 tablespoons lemon juice

½ cup (4 fl oz/125 ml) boiling water

3 tablespoons sugar

2 tablespoons light corn syrup

Chocolate Sauce

⅔ cup (5 oz/155 g) sugar

½ cup (4 fl oz/125 ml) nonfat milk

¼ cup (¾ oz/20 g) unsweetened
  Dutch-process cocoa

1½ tablespoons cornstarch (corn flour)

1 teaspoon vanilla extract (essence)

Preparation: 25 minutes ✳ Cooking: 40 minutes ✳ Serves 4

Choose slightly underripe, firm pears for this autumn dessert as overly soft fruit may turn mushy during cooking. Pears are a good source of vitamins A and C. In addition to the preparation time, allow at least 20 minutes for the pears to chill before serving.

✳ Preheat an oven to 350°F (180°C).

✳ In a 13-by-9-by-2-inch (33-by-23-by-5-cm) baking dish, arrange the pears, cut side down, and top with the lemon juice.

✳ In a small bowl, combine the water, sugar and corn syrup and stir to mix well. Pour over the pears. Cover the dish with aluminum foil and bake until the pears are tender when pierced with a fork, 25–35 minutes. Cool in the pan for 10 minutes.

✳ Using a slotted spoon, transfer the pears to a container, cover and refrigerate for 20 minutes to 8 hours. Discard the syrup.

✳ To serve, slice each pear half lengthwise into thin slices, without cutting all the way through the stem end, place 2 halves on each dessert plate and press down gently to form fans. Top each with 1 tablespoon of the chocolate sauce.

Chocolate Sauce

✳ In a small saucepan over medium heat, combine the sugar, milk, cocoa and cornstarch. Simmer, stirring constantly with a wire whisk, until the mixture thickens, about 5 minutes. Remove from the heat and stir in the vanilla. Store in an airtight container in the refrigerator for up to 1 week. One serving is 1 tablespoon.

Nutritional Analysis per Serving

Calories 308 (Kilojoules 1,295); Total fat 2g; Saturated fat 1g; Protein 3g; Cholesterol 1mg; Carbohydrates 76g; Sodium 62mg; Dietary fiber 4g; Calories from fat 5%

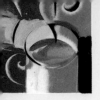

¼ cup (2 oz/60 g) sugar

1 cup (8 fl oz/250 ml) water

1 vanilla bean (pod), split lengthwise

1 cup (6 oz/185 g) cantaloupe
   (rock melon) cubes

1 cup (6 oz/185 g) honeydew cubes

1 cup (4 oz/125 g) blueberries

¼ cup (⅓ oz/10 g) chopped fresh mint

4 fresh mint sprigs

Shopping Tip

You'll find whole vanilla beans in jars in the spice section of most markets. If you can't find them, substitute 1 teaspoon vanilla extract (essence). Stir it into the cooked syrup.

Melon and Blueberries in Sauce

Preparation: 20 minutes ✳ Cooking: 35 minutes ✳ Serves 4

In addition to the preparation and cooking times, you'll need to allow 2 hours for chilling before serving. Melons, blueberries and mint— summertime favorites—are all rich in vitamins A and C, so enjoy this colorful dessert knowing it's both good and good for you.

✳ To make the syrup, in a small saucepan over medium heat, dissolve the sugar in the water. Scrape the seeds from the vanilla bean and add the seeds and bean to the pan. Reduce the heat to low and simmer, stirring constantly, until the syrup is hot, about 3 minutes. Remove from the heat and let steep for 30 minutes.

✳ Strain the syrup through a fine-mesh sieve and discard the vanilla bean and seeds.

✳ In a large bowl, combine the melon cubes, blueberries and chopped mint. Add the strained syrup and toss to coat well. Cover and refrigerate for at least 2 hours.

✳ To serve, divide among 4 individual dessert dishes and top with the mint sprigs. Serve chilled or at room temperature.

Nutritional Analysis per Serving

Calories 106 (Kilojoules 444); Total fat 0g; Saturated fat 0g; Protein 1g; Cholesterol 0mg; Carbohydrates 26g; Sodium 10mg; Dietary fiber 1g; Calories from fat 2%

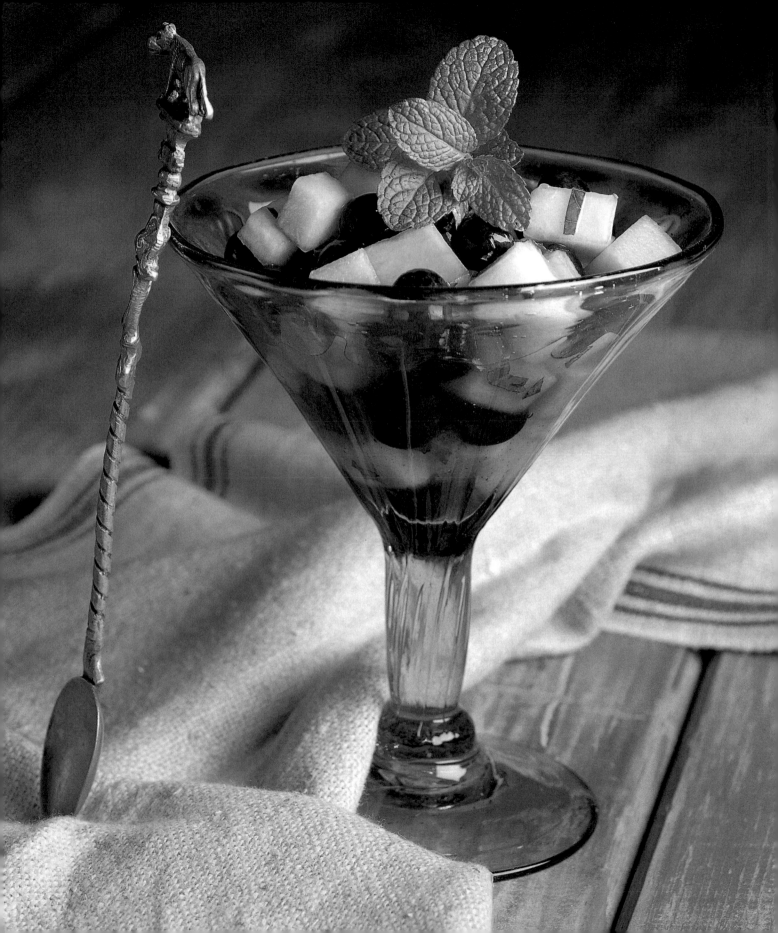

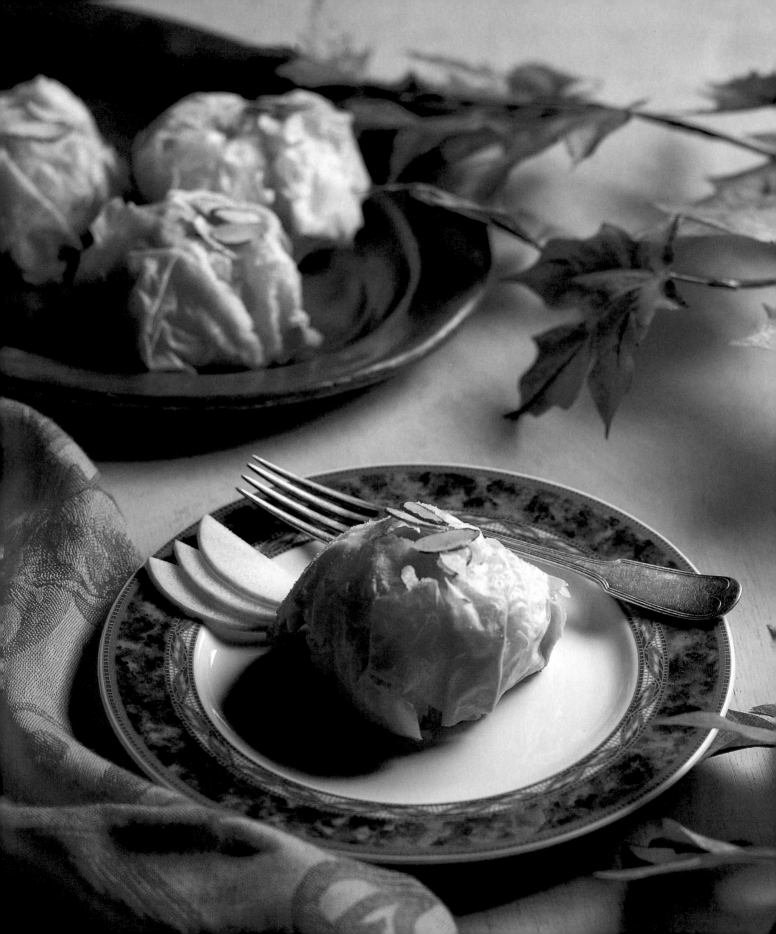

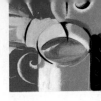

Baked Apples

4 tart apples, such as Granny Smith,
    peeled and cored

2 tablespoons lemon juice

2 tablespoons chopped almonds

1 tablespoon firmly packed
    brown sugar

2 teaspoons margarine

½ teaspoon ground cinnamon

½ teaspoon vanilla extract (essence)

4 sheets frozen filo pastry, thawed,
    unfolded and stacked

1 egg white

2 tablespoons sliced (flaked) almonds

2 teaspoons sugar

Preparation: 25 minutes ✳ Cooking: 40 minutes ✳ Serves 4

Wrapped apples can be prepared up to 2 days ahead. Just assemble, cover with plastic wrap and refrigerate, then bake before serving. Frozen filo pastry can be thawed, wrapped airtight, in the refrigerator for 8 hours or overnight. To prevent the pastry sheets from drying out and becoming brittle, cover them with plastic wrap or waxed paper and a damp towel while you prepare the apples.

✳ Preheat an oven to 350°F (180°C). Coat a shallow glass baking dish with nonstick cooking spray. Brush the apples with the lemon juice.

✳ In a small bowl, mix together the chopped almonds, brown sugar, margarine, cinnamon and vanilla. Spoon an equal amount of the mixture into the hollowed-out cores of each apple.

✳ Using a sharp knife, cut the stacked filo sheets into quarters. Place an apple, base side down, onto the center of each stack and bring up the edges and tuck the ends into the hollowed-out core.

✳ Place the wrapped apples, seam side down, in the prepared dish and brush with the egg white. Top with the sliced almonds and sprinkle with the sugar. Bake until the pastry is golden, 35–40 minutes.

✳ To serve, divide among 4 individual dessert plates.

Nutritional Analysis per Serving

Calories 219 (Kilojoules 920); Total fat 7g; Saturated fat 1g; Protein 4g; Cholesterol 0mg; Carbohydrates 37g; Sodium 132mg; Dietary fiber 3g; Calories from fat 29%

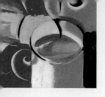

2½ cups (10 oz/315 g) raspberries

1 cup (8 fl oz/250 ml) nonfat milk

¼ cup (2 oz/60 g) sugar

4 fresh mint sprigs

Raspberry Sherbet

Preparation: 20 minutes ✳ *Chilling: 2 hours* ✳ *Serves 4*

✳ In a blender, combine the raspberries, milk and sugar and process until smooth.

✳ Pour into a 13-by-9-by-2-inch (33-by-23-by-5-cm) baking dish. Cover and freeze until firm, about 2 hours.

✳ Return the sherbet to the blender in batches and process until smooth. Freeze in the baking dish until ready to serve.

✳ To serve, divide among 4 individual dessert dishes. Garnish each with a mint sprig.

Nutritional Analysis per Serving

Calories 111 (Kilojoules 468); Total fat 1g; Saturated fat 0g; Protein 3g; Cholesterol 1mg; Carbohydrates 25g; Sodium 32mg; Dietary fiber 3g; Calories from fat 4%

1½ cups (12 fl oz/375 ml) orange juice

2½ cups (10 oz/315 g) blueberries

1½ cups (12 fl oz/375 ml) lowfat buttermilk

¼ cup (2 oz/60 g) sugar

¼ cup (2 fl oz/60 ml) lemon juice

1 teaspoon finely grated lemon zest

8 fresh mint sprigs

Lemon-Blueberry Ice Milk

Preparation: 20 minutes ✳ *Chilling: 2 hours* ✳ *Serves 8*

✳ In a blender, combine the orange juice, 2 cups (8 oz/250 g) of blueberries, the buttermilk, sugar and lemon juice and zest and process until smooth.

✳ Pour into a 13-by-9-by-2-inch (33-by-23-by-5-cm) baking dish. Cover and freeze until firm, about 2 hours.

✳ Return the ice milk to the blender in batches and process until smooth. Freeze in the baking dish until ready to serve.

✳ To serve, divide among 8 individual dessert dishes. Top each with an equal amount of the remaining berries. Garnish each with a mint sprig.

Nutritional Analysis per Serving

Calories 93 (Kilojoules 390); Total fat 1g; Saturated fat 0g; Protein 2g; Cholesterol 3mg; Carbohydrates 20g; Sodium 70mg; Dietary fiber 1g; Calories from fat 6%

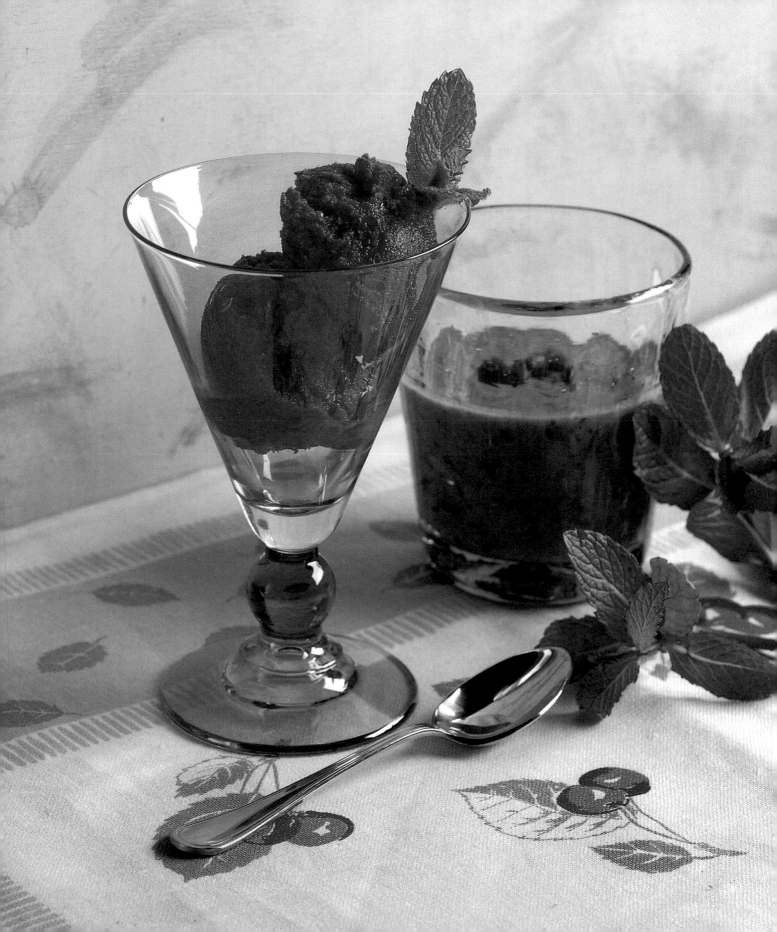

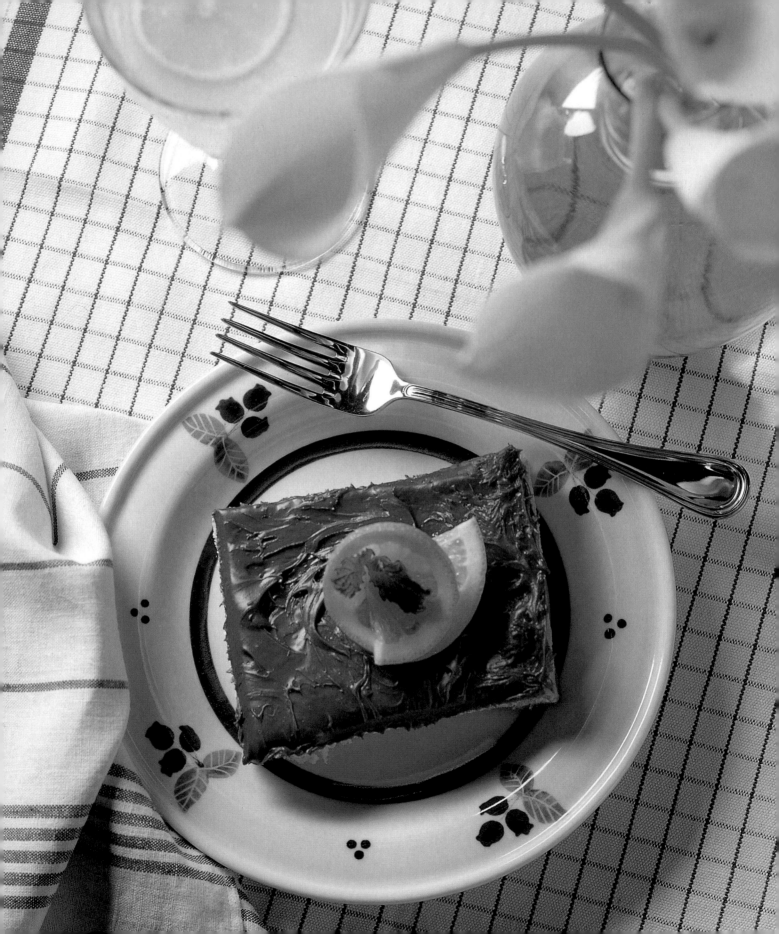

Sponge Cake with Chocolate-Orange Frosting

Preparation: 35 minutes ✳ *Cooking: 20 minutes* ✳ *Serves 16*

1 cup (3 oz/90 g) sifted cake
  (soft-wheat) flour

1 teaspoon baking powder

⅛ teaspoon salt

3 eggs, separated

1 cup (8 oz/250 g) sugar

2 teaspoons vanilla extract (essence)

¼ cup (2 fl oz/60 ml) water

2 egg whites

Chocolate-Orange Frosting

3 cups (12 oz/375 g) confectioners'
  (icing) sugar, sifted

⅓ cup (1 oz/30 g) unsweetened
  Dutch-process cocoa

¼ cup (2 fl oz/60 ml) boiling water

2 tablespoons margarine

½ teaspoon vanilla extract (essence)

½ teaspoon orange extract (essence)

Cooking Tip

✳ For a different-flavored frosting, substitute almond, lemon or additional vanilla extract for the orange extract.

✳ Preheat an oven to 350°F (180°C). Coat a 13-by-9-by-2-inch (33-by-23-by-5-cm) baking pan with nonstick cooking spray.

✳ In a small bowl, combine the flour, baking powder and salt.

✳ In a large bowl, using an electric mixer on high speed, beat the 3 egg yolks for 1 minute. With the mixer on high speed, gradually beat in ¾ cup (6 oz/185 g) of the sugar. Continue beating on high speed until the mixture is thick and the yolks are pale, about 3 minutes.

✳ With the mixer on medium speed, beat in the vanilla and water. With the mixer on low speed, gradually add the dry ingredients and beat until blended.

✳ In another large bowl, using an electric mixer on high speed and clean beaters, beat the 5 egg whites until foamy. Continuing to beat on high speed, gradually add the remaining sugar until stiff peaks form.

✳ Stir ½ cup (4 fl oz/125 ml) of the egg white mixture into the egg yolk–flour mixture. Fold in the remaining egg whites.

✳ Pour into the prepared pan and bake until the cake springs back when pressed in the center, about 20 minutes. Cool in the pan. When the cake is cool, spread the top with the Chocolate-Orange Frosting.

✳ To serve, slice into 16 pieces and divide among individual dessert plates. Store wrapped in plastic wrap in the refrigerator for up to 3 days.

Chocolate-Orange Frosting

✳ In a large bowl, combine the confectioners' sugar, cocoa powder, water, margarine and extracts. Using an electric mixer on high speed, beat until smooth.

Nutritional Analysis per Serving

Calories 194 (Kilojoules 814); Total fat 3g; Saturated fat 1g; Protein 2g; Cholesterol 40mg; Carbohydrates 41g; Sodium 96mg; Dietary fiber 0g; Calories from fat 13%

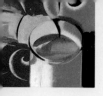

2 cantaloupes (rock melons), halved
  and seeded

4 egg whites

¼ cup (2 oz/60 g) sugar

1 teaspoon vanilla extract (essence)

2 cups (16 fl oz/500 ml) Raspberry
  Sherbet (recipe on page 224)

Nutrition Tip

✱ Cantaloupe is an outstanding source
of vitamins A and C, with one serving
providing more than half of the recommended daily allowance of A and more
than 100 percent of C. It also offers a lot
of the antioxidant beta-carotene, along
with ample fiber and B vitamins.

Meringue-Topped Cantaloupe

Preparation: 25 minutes ✱ *Cooking: 25 minutes* ✱ *Serves 4*

*Meringues must be fully cooked to eliminate the risks associated with
raw eggs. They will appear golden brown on top and completely set in
the middle. Store leftover meringues in an airtight container at room
temperature for up to 3 days.*

✱ Preheat an oven to 300°F (150°C). Coat a large baking sheet
with nonstick cooking spray.

✱ Using a melon baller, make balls from the 4 cantaloupe
halves, reserving the shells. Slice the bottom of each shell so that
it stands upright.

✱ In a large bowl, using an electric mixer on high speed, beat
the egg whites until soft peaks form. While continuing to beat on
high speed, gradually add the sugar until stiff peaks form. Gently
fold in the vanilla.

✱ Spoon the meringue onto the prepared baking sheet, forming
4 rounds of the same diameter as the cantaloupe shells. Bake
until golden brown and set in the center, 20–25 minutes.

✱ To serve, place the cantaloupe shells on 4 individual plates, place
an equal amount of the melon balls and sherbet into each shell.
Top each with a meringue.

Nutritional Analysis per Serving

Calories 282 (Kilojoules 1,184); Total fat 1g; Saturated fat 0g; Protein 9g;
Cholesterol 1mg; Carbohydrates 63g; Sodium 111mg; Dietary fiber 5g;
Calories from fat 4%

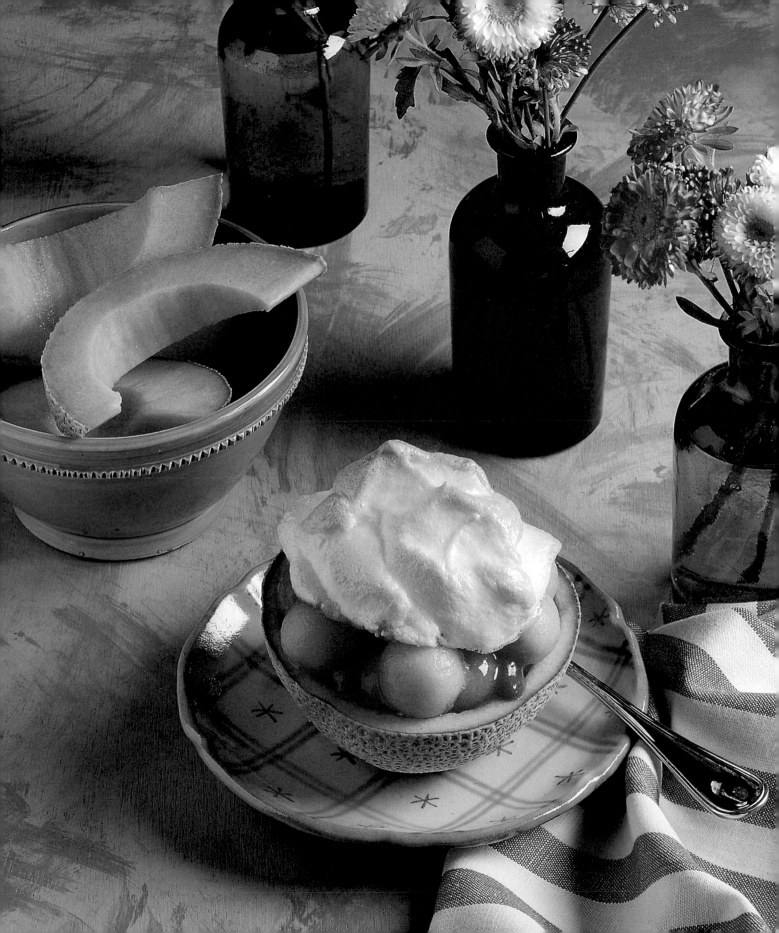

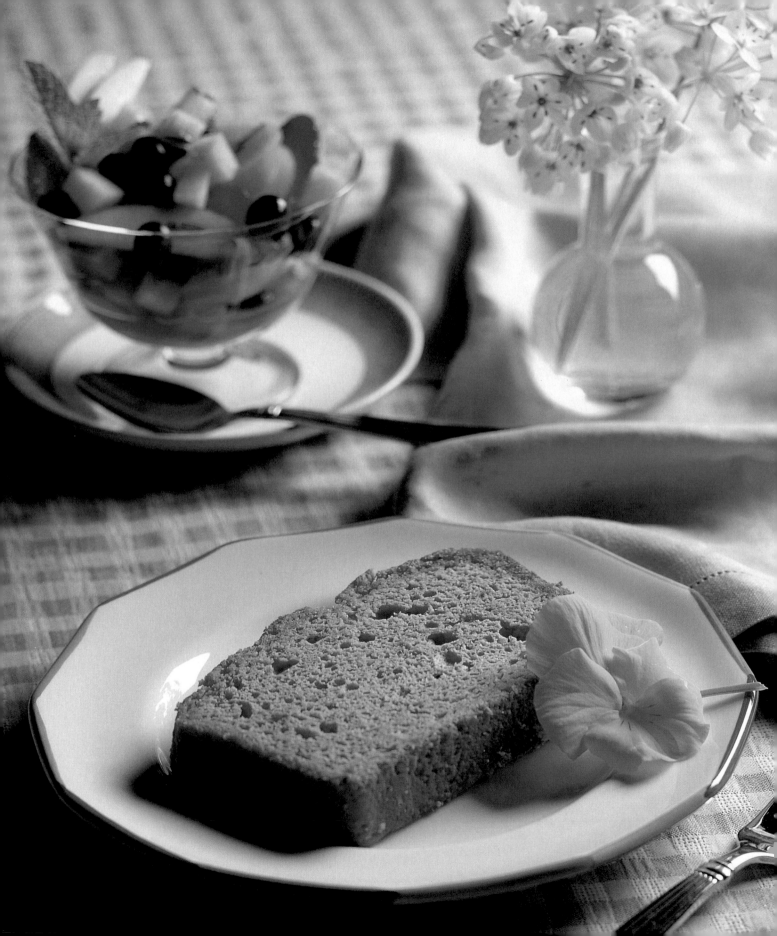

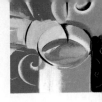

2 peaches or nectarines, peeled,
    pitted and sliced
1 cup (4 oz/125 g) blueberries
1 cup (4 oz/125 g) strawberries
1 cup (6 oz/185 g) cantaloupe
    (rock melon) chunks
1 cup (6 oz/185 g) honeydew or
    watermelon chunks
1 kiwifruit, peeled and sliced
2 tablespoons honey
¼ cup (2 fl oz/60 ml) orange juice
3 tablespoons chopped fresh mint
1 tablespoon lemon juice

2½ cups (12½ oz/390 g) unbleached
    flour
2 teaspoons baking powder
½ teaspoon baking soda
    (bicarbonate of soda)
1½ teaspoons ground cinnamon
¼ teaspoon ground nutmeg
¼ teaspoon ground cloves
¼ teaspoon salt
¼ cup (2 oz/60 g) margarine
¾ cup (6 oz/185 ml) sugar
½ cup (3½ oz/105 g) firmly packed
    brown sugar
2 eggs
1 egg white
1⅞ cups (15 oz/470 g) pumpkin purée
⅓ cup (3 oz/90 g) plus 2 tablespoons
    nonfat plain yogurt

Honey-Mint Fruit Compote

Preparation: 15 minutes ✴ Chilling: 30 minutes ✴ Serves 4

✴ In a large bowl, combine the peaches or nectarines, blueberries, strawberries, cantaloupe, honeydew or watermelon and kiwifruit. In a small bowl, whisk together the honey, orange juice, mint and lemon juice.

✴ Spoon the honey mixture over the fruit, cover with plastic wrap and refrigerate to allow the flavors to marry, at least 30 minutes.

✴ To serve, divide among 4 individual bowls. Serve chilled.

Nutritional Analysis per Serving

Calories 134 (Kilojoules 564); Total fat 1g; Saturated fat 0g; Protein 2g; Cholesterol 0mg; Carbohydrates 34g; Sodium 12mg; Dietary fiber 4g; Calories from fat 3%

Pumpkin Spice Bread

Preparation: 20 minutes ✴ Cooking: 1 hour ✴ Serves 8

✴ Preheat an oven to 350°F (180°C). Coat a 9-by-5-inch (23-by-13-cm) loaf pan with nonstick cooking spray.

✴ In a medium bowl, combine the flour, baking powder, baking soda, cinnamon, nutmeg, cloves and salt. In a large bowl, using an electric mixer or by hand, beat the margarine and sugars until creamy. Add the eggs and egg white and beat until blended. Add the pumpkin and yogurt and beat until smooth. Gradually add the flour mixture and beat until blended.

✴ Pour the batter into the prepared loaf pan and bake until a toothpick inserted in the center comes out clean, about 1 hour. Cool in the pan for 10 minutes.

✴ To serve, cut into 8 slices and place on individual plates. Store in an airtight container at room temperature for up to 2 days.

Nutritional Analysis per Serving

Calories 389 (Kilojoules 1,634); Total fat 8g; Saturated fat 1g; Protein 8g; Cholesterol 53mg; Carbohydrates 73g; Sodium 374mg; Dietary fiber 2g; Calories from fat 18%

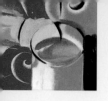

1½ cups (12 fl oz/375 ml) nonfat milk

¼ cup (2 oz/60 g) plus 2 tablespoons
sugar

2 teaspoons finely grated orange zest

½ teaspoon finely grated lemon zest

1 teaspoon vanilla extract (essence)

¼ teaspoon salt

4 egg yolks

Raspberry Sauce

2½ cups (10 oz/315 g) raspberries

2 tablespoons confectioners'
(icing) sugar

2 tablespoons cold water

2 teaspoons cornstarch (cornflour)

Orange Custard with Raspberry Sauce

Preparation: 20 minutes ✶ Cooking: 1 hour 10 minutes ✶ Serves 4

You need to do some advance planning to serve this dessert because it takes over an hour to cook and needs another hour to chill. However, the preparation is fairly quick and the taste worth the effort. This custard is a good choice for a dinner party as it can be done ahead and the presentation will impress your guests.

✶ Preheat an oven to 325°F (165°C).

✶ In a medium bowl, combine the milk, sugar, orange and lemon zest, vanilla, salt and egg yolks and whisk until blended.

✶ Divide among four ¾-cup (6–fl oz/180-ml) custard cups. Place the cups in a shallow baking dish and add enough hot water to reach 1 inch (2.5 cm) up the sides of the cups.

✶ Bake until a knife inserted in the center comes out clean (the center will still jiggle a little), 1 hour 10 minutes. Cool completely before serving, about 1 hour.

✶ To serve, top each custard with an equal amount of the Raspberry Sauce.

Raspberry Sauce

✶ Press the raspberries through a fine-mesh sieve into a small saucepan to remove the seeds. Place the pan with the resulting purée and juice over medium heat, add the confectioners' sugar and simmer for 2 minutes. In a small jar, combine the water and cornstarch and shake to mix well. Add to the raspberries and simmer, stirring frequently, until the sauce has thickened, about 3 minutes. Remove from the heat and cool before serving. One serving is 3 tablespoons.

Nutritional Analysis per Serving

Calories 224 (Kilojoules 939); Total fat 6g; Saturated fat 2g; Protein 7g; Cholesterol 214mg; Carbohydrates 37g; Sodium 190mg; Dietary fiber 3g; Calories from fat 23%

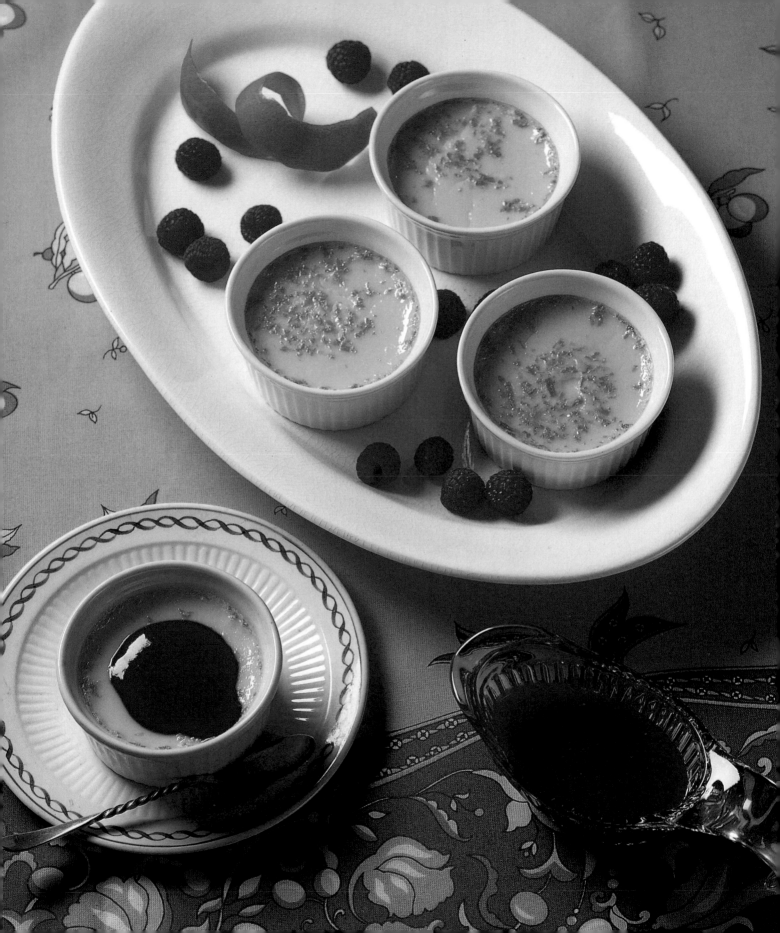

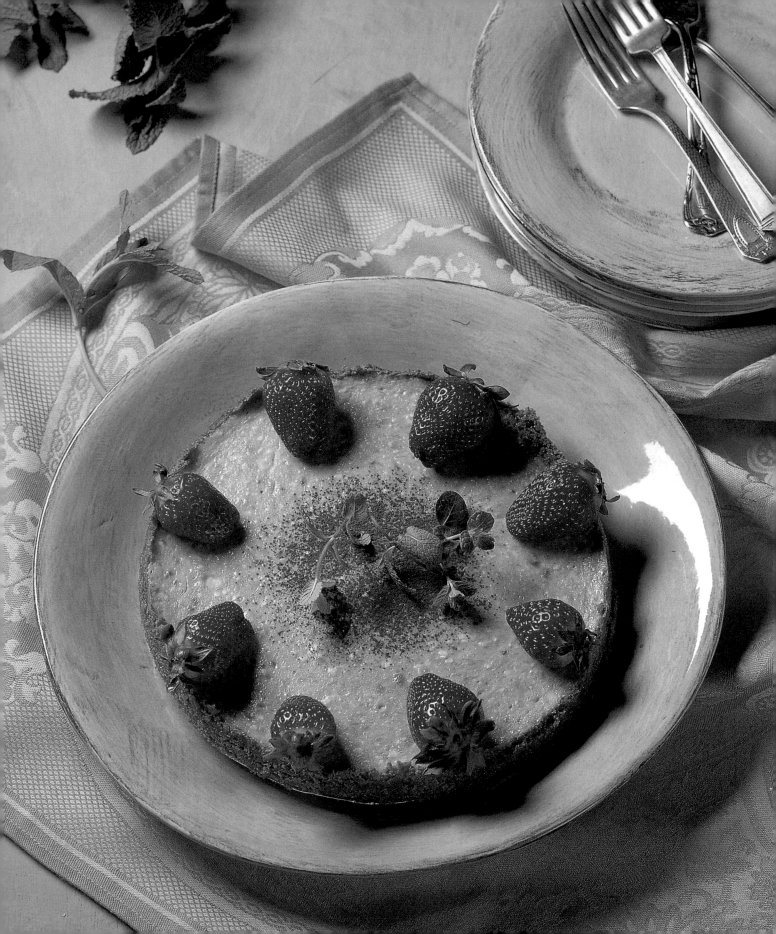

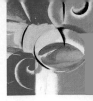

Banana Cheesecake

½ cup (1½ oz/45 g) plus 2 tablespoons
  graham cracker crumbs

2 tablespoons plus ½ cup (4 oz/125 g)
  sugar

2 tablespoons margarine, melted

4 large bananas, mashed

8 oz (250 g) nonfat cream cheese

½ cup (4 oz/125 g) nonfat small curd
  cottage cheese

1 egg

2 teaspoons vanilla extract (essence)

½ teaspoon sweetened cocoa

8 strawberries

8 fresh mint sprigs

Preparation: 25 minutes ✳ *Cooking: 1 hour* ✳ *Serves 8*

In addition to the preparation and cooking times, allow at least 1 hour and 15 minutes for the cake to cool before serving. Ask your guests what the secret ingredient is in this dessert and few will guess that it's cottage cheese! The bananas and cottage cheese replace most of the cream cheese— and its fat—found in traditional cheesecakes. Bananas also supply vitamins, niacin and potassium.

✳ Preheat an oven to 300°F (150°C). Coat the bottom and sides of a 9-inch (23-cm) springform pan with nonstick cooking spray.

✳ To make the crust, in a medium bowl, combine the graham cracker crumbs, 2 tablespoons sugar and margarine and stir to mix well. Lightly press the mixture into the bottom of the prepared pan.

✳ To make the filling, in a food processor with the metal blade or in a blender, combine the bananas, cream cheese, cottage cheese, egg, vanilla and ½ cup (4 oz/125 g) sugar and process until smooth.

✳ Pour the filling into the crust and bake until the center is set, about 1 hour. Turn off the oven, prop open the oven door and leave the cake in the oven to cool for 15 minutes. Remove the cake from the oven and cool completely in the pan, about 1 hour.

✳ To serve, release the cake from the pan, sprinkle the top with the cocoa, slice into 8 wedges and divide among individual dessert plates. Garnish each wedge with a strawberry and a mint sprig. Store covered in the refrigerator for up to 4 days.

Nutritional Analysis per Serving

Calories 236 (Kilojoules 993); Total fat 5g; Saturated fat 1g; Protein 8g; Cholesterol 31mg; Carbohydrates 41g; Sodium 284mg; Dietary fiber 1g; Calories from fat 18%

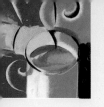

½ cup (1½ oz/45 g) plus 2 tablespoons
  graham cracker crumbs
2 tablespoons plus ¾ cup
  (6 oz/185 g) sugar
2 tablespoons margarine, melted
2 cups (1 lb/500 g) nonfat
  ricotta cheese
8 oz (250 g) nonfat cream cheese
1 egg
1½ teaspoons vanilla extract (essence)
⅓ cup (1 oz/30 g) unsweetened
  Dutch-process cocoa
3 tablespoons all-purpose flour
1½ oz (45 g) semisweet (plain)
  chocolate, melted and cooled
½ cup (4 oz/125 g) nonfat
  vanilla yogurt
3 tablespoons nonfat dairy sour cream
¼ oz (7 g) semisweet (plain)
  chocolate, grated

Chocolate Cheesecake

Preparation: 25 minutes ✳ Cooking: 1 hour ✳ Serves 8

In addition to the preparation and cooking times, allow at least 1 hour and 15 minutes for the cake to cool before serving. This cake satisfies even the most serious "chocoholic." The chocolate makes the cake sweeter than plain versions, but it is still not so sweet that fans of more tangy cheese-cakes won't enjoy it.

✳ Preheat an oven to 300°F (150°C). Coat the bottom and sides of a 9-inch (23-cm) springform pan with nonstick cooking spray.

✳ To make the crust, in a medium bowl, combine the graham cracker crumbs, 2 tablespoons sugar and margarine and stir to mix well. Lightly press the mixture into the bottom of the prepared pan.

✳ To make the filling, in a food processor with the metal blade or in a blender, combine the ricotta, cream cheese and ¾ cup (6 oz/185 g) sugar and process until smooth. Add the egg and vanilla and process until blended. Gradually add the cocoa, flour and melted chocolate and process until smooth.

✳ Pour the filling into the crust and bake until the center is set, about 1 hour. Turn off the oven, prop open the oven door and leave the cake in the oven to cool for 15 minutes. Remove the cake from the oven and cool completely in the pan, about 1 hour.

✳ To make the icing, in a small bowl, combine the yogurt and sour cream and stir to mix well.

✳ To serve, release from the pan, top with a thin layer of the icing and grated chocolate, slice into 8 wedges and divide among individual dessert plates. Store covered in the refrigerator for up to 4 days.

Nutritional Analysis per Serving

Calories 297 (Kilojoules 1,247); Total fat 7g; Saturated fat 2g; Protein 16g; Cholesterol 30mg; Carbohydrates 42g; Sodium 344mg; Dietary fiber 0g; Calories from fat 21%

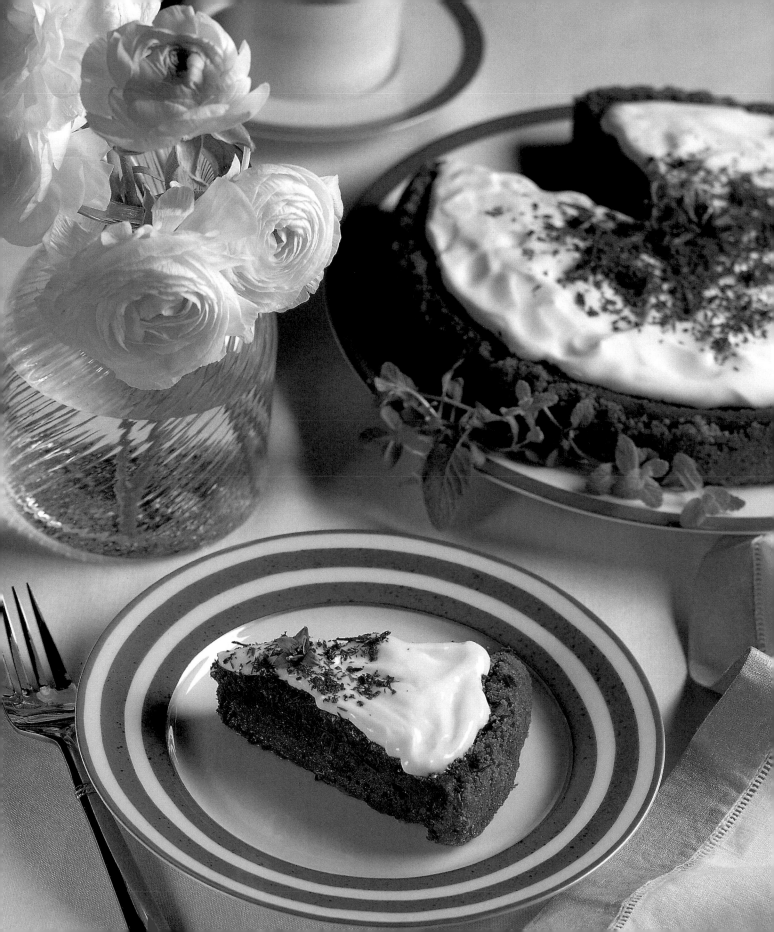

Index

Tips

Resources Guide

The following Jane Fonda video and audio programs optimally complement Cooking for Healthy Living:

✳ **Abs, Buns & Thighs**
Two 25-minute low impact aerobic and toning programs to be used alternately.

✳ **Low Impact Aerobics & Stretch**
A 25-minute aerobic and 20-minute stretch and relaxation routine.

✳ **Total Body Sculpting**
Two 25-minute toning workouts to be used alternately.

✳ **Favorite Fat Burners**
A 50-minute compilation of Jane's favorite aerobic routines, plus her personal 15-minute nutritional program.

✳ **Complete Workout**
Thirty-five minutes of low impact aerobics and 35-minutes of full body sculpting and stretching.

✳ **Yoga Exercise Workout**
A 50-minute, three-part workout of modified yoga postures.

✳ **Fitness Walkout Audio**
Two hours of energetic music with Jane's motivational guidelines to keep you moving at an aerobic pace.

For a catalog of Jane Fonda exercise videos and audio cassettes:
✳ Jane Fonda Workout
P.O. Box 22
Lake Oswego, OR 97034
800 824-7148

To order The Famine Within *video:*
✳ Direct Cinema Limited
P.O. Box 10003
Santa Monica, CA 90410
800 525-0000

To mail order herbs and spices:
✳ Penzeys, Limited
P.O. Box 1448
Waukesha, WI 53187
414 574-0277

For information on obtaining organic produce:
✳ Community Supported
Agriculture West
1156 High Street
Santa Cruz, CA 95064
408 459-3964

✳ Community Supported Agriculture
of North America
RR3, Box 85 Jugend Road
Great Barrington, MA 01230

For information on obtaining bison:
✳ North American Bison Cooperative
RR1, Box 162 B
New Rockford, ND 58356
701 947-2505, fax 701 947-2105

For referrals on eating disorder treatment:
✳ National Association of Anorexia
Nervosa and Associated Disorders
P.O. Box 7
Highland Park, IL 60035
847 831-3438

✳ National Eating Disorders
Organization
6655 South Yale Avenue
Tulsa, OK 74136
918 481-4044

✳ International Association of
Eating Disorders Professionals
123 NW 13th Street, Suite 206
Boca Raton, FL 33432
407 338-6494

✳ National Eating Disorder
Information Centre
200 Elizabeth Street
Toronto, ON Canada M5G 2C4
416 340-4156

Acknowledgments

For Weldon Owen: Vice President and Publisher: Wendely Harvey; Managing Editor: Jill Fox; Consulting Editor: Norman Kolpas; Recipe Analysis and Nutritional Consultant: Hill Nutrition Associates, Inc; Recipe Writer: Robin Vitetta; Recipe Contributor: Karen Averitt; Eating Disorders Consultant: Janice M. Cauwels, Ph.D; Consultants: Julie LaFond and Nancy Howitt; Editorial Concept: Lu Sierra; Copy Editor: Judith Dunham; Design Concept: John Bull; Designer: Kari Perin; Production Director: Stephanie Sherman; Production Coordinator: Tarji Mickelson; Production Editors: Ruth Jacobson and Janique Gascoigne; Editorial Assistant: Sara Deseran; Proofreaders: Desne Border and Ken DellaPenta; Indexer: ALTA Indexing Service; Illustrator: Jennie Oppenheimer; Recipe Testers: Peggy Fallon and Paul Torgerson; Food Photographer: Joyce Oudkerk Pool; Food Stylist: Pouké; Assistant Food Stylist: Michelle Syracuse; Prop Stylist: Carol Hacker; Photography Assistant: Myriam Varela; Photographer, cover and pages 9, 12 and 20: Firooz Zahedi; Stylists, cover and pages 9 and 12: Chris McMillan (hair), Wayne Massarelli (cover and page 12 makeup), Lutz (page 9 makeup), Linda Medevene (clothing); Photographer, page 11: John Engstead; Photographer, page 28: Rob Lewine; Food Props: American Rag, Cyclamen Studio and Gibson Scheid.